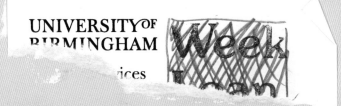

NINTH EDITION

RESPIRATORY PHYSIOLOGY

THE ESSENTIALS

15

NINTH EDITION

RESPIRATORY PHYSIOLOGY

THE ESSENTIALS

John B. West, M.D., Ph.D., D.Sc.

Professor of Medicine and Physiology
University of California, San Diego
School of Medicine
La Jolla, California

Wolters Kluwer | Lippincott Williams & Wilkins
Health
Philadelphia · Baltimore · New York · London
Buenos Aires · Hong Kong · Sydney · Tokyo

Acquisitions Editor: Crystal Taylor
Product Manager: Catherine Noonan
Marketing Manager: Joy Fisher-Williams
Vendor Manager: Bridgett Dougherty
Manufacturing Manager: Margie Orzech
Designer: Holly Reid McLaughlin
Compositor: SPi Global

Ninth Edition

Printed in China

351 West Camden Street   Two Commerce Square
Baltimore, MD 21201   2001 Market Street
                                           Philadelphia, PA 19103

First Edition, 1974
Second Edition, 1982
Third Edition, 1987
Fourth Edition, 1992
Fifth Edition, 1998
Sixth Edition, 2003
Seventh Edition, 2004
Eighth Edition, 2008

The publisher is not responsible (as a matter of product liability, negligence, or otherwise) for any injury resulting from any material contained herein. This publication contains information relating to general principles of medical care that should not be construed as specific instructions for individual patients. Manufacturers' product information and package inserts should be reviewed for current information, including contraindications, dosages, and precautions.

Library of Congress Cataloging-in-Publication Data
West, John B. (John Burnard)
Respiratory physiology : the essentials / John B. West. — 9th ed.
    p. ; cm.
Includes index.
ISBN 978-1-60913-640-6
1. Respiration. I. Title.
[DNLM: 1. Respiratory Physiological Phenomena. WF 102]
QP121.W43   2012
612.2—dc23

2011019298

DISCLAIMER
Care has been taken to confirm the accuracy of the information present and to describe generally accepted practices. However, the authors, editors, and publisher are not responsible for errors or omissions or for any consequences from application of the information in this book and make no warranty, expressed or implied, with respect to the currency, completeness, or accuracy of the contents of the publication. Application of this information in a particular situation remains the professional responsibility of the practitioner; the clinical treatments described and recommended may not be considered absolute and universal recommendations.

The authors, editors, and publisher have exerted every effort to ensure that drug selection and dosage set forth in this text are in accordance with the current recommendations and practice at the time of publication. However, in view of ongoing research, changes in government regulations, and the constant flow of information relating to drug therapy and drug reactions, the reader is urged to check the package insert for each drug for any change in indications and dosage and for added warnings and precautions. This is particularly important when the recommended agent is a new or infrequently employed drug.

Some drugs and medical devices presented in this publication have Food and Drug Administration (FDA) clearance for limited use in restricted research settings. It is the responsibility of the health care provider to ascertain the FDA status of each drug or device planned for use in their clinical practice.

To purchase additional copies of this book, call our customer service department at (800) 638-3030 or fax orders to (301) 223-2320. International customers should call (301) 223-2300.

Visit Lippincott Williams & Wilkins on the Internet: http://www.lww.com. Lippincott Williams & Wilkins customer service representatives are available from 8:30 am to 6:00 PM, EST.

9 8 7 6 5 4 3 2 1

To P.H.W.

Preface

This book first appeared some 35 years ago, and it has been well received and translated into over 15 languages. It is appropriate to briefly review the objectives.

First, the book is intended as an introductory text for medical students and allied health students. As such, it will normally be used in conjunction with a course of lectures, and this is the case at University of California, San Diego (UCSD) School of Medicine. Indeed, the first edition was written because I believed that there was no appropriate textbook at that time to accompany the first-year physiology course.

Second, the book is written as a review for residents and fellows in such areas as pulmonary medicine, anesthesiology, and internal medicine, particularly to help them prepare for licensing and other examinations. Here the requirements are somewhat different. The reader is familiar with the general area but needs to have his or her memory jogged on various points, and the many didactic diagrams are particularly important.

It might be useful to add a word or two about how the book meshes with the lectures to the first-year medical students at UCSD. We are limited to about twelve 50-minute lectures on respiratory physiology supplemented by two laboratories and three discussion groups. The lectures follow the individual chapters of the book closely, with most chapters corresponding to a single lecture. The exceptions are that Chapter 5 has two lectures (one on normal gas exchange, hypoventilation, and shunt; another on the difficult topic of ventilation-perfusion relationships); Chapter 6 has two lectures (one on blood-gas transport and another on acid-base balance); Chapter 7 has two lectures (on statics and dynamics); and if the schedule of the course allows, the section on polluted atmospheres in Chapter 9 is expanded to include an additional lecture on defense systems of the lung. There is no lecture on Chapter 10, "Tests of Pulmonary Function," because this is not part of the core course. It is included partly for interest and partly because of its importance to people who work in pulmonary function laboratories.

Several colleagues have suggested that Chapter 6 on gas transport should come earlier in the book because knowledge of the oxygen dissociation curve is needed to properly understand diffusion across the blood-gas barrier. In fact, we make this switch in our lecture course. However, the various chapters of the book can stand alone, and I prefer the present ordering of chapters because it leads to a nice flow of ideas as the cartoons at the beginning of each chapter indicate. The order of chapters also probably makes it easier for the reader who is reviewing material.

It is sometimes argued that Chapter 7, "Mechanics of Breathing," should come earlier, for example, with Chapter 2, "Ventilation." My experience of over 40 years of teaching is against this. The topic of mechanics is so complex and difficult for the present-day medical student that it is best dealt with separately and later in the course when the students are more prepared for the concepts. Parenthetically, it seems that many modern medical students find concepts of pressure, flow, and resistance much more difficult than was the case 25 years ago, whereas, of course, they breeze through any discussion of molecular biology.

Some colleagues have recommended that more space should be devoted to sample calculations using the equations in the text and various clinical examples. My belief is that these topics are well suited to the lectures or discussion groups, which can then embellish the basic information. Indeed, if the calculations and clinical examples were included in the book, there would be precious little to talk about. Many of the questions at the end of each chapter require calculations.

The present edition has been updated in a number of areas, including the control of ventilation, physiology of high altitude, the pulmonary circulation, and forced expiration. A new section includes discussions of the answers to the questions in Appendix B. A major change in the previous edition was the addition of animations and other Web-based material to help explain some of the most difficult concepts. The section of the text that the animations refer to is indicated by the symbol 📷 .

Heroic efforts have been made to keep the book lean, in spite of enormous temptations to fatten it. Occasionally, medical students wonder if the book is too superficial. I disagree; in fact, if pulmonary fellows beginning their training in intensive care units fully understood all the material on gas exchange and mechanics, the world would be a better place.

Many students and teachers have written to query statements in the book or to make suggestions for improvement. I respond personally to every point that is raised and much appreciate this input.

John West
jwest@ucsd.edu

Contents

Structure and Function

▶ **HOW THE ARCHITECTURE OF THE LUNG SUBSERVES ITS FUNCTION**

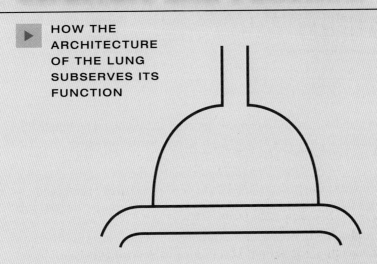

We begin with a short review of the relationships between structure and function in the lung. First, we look at the blood-gas interface, where the exchange of the respiratory gases occurs. Next we look at how oxygen is brought to the interface through the airways and then how the blood removes the oxygen from the lung. Finally, two potential problems of the lung are briefly addressed: how the alveoli maintain their stability and how the lung is kept clean in a polluted environment.

The lung is for gas exchange. Its prime function is to allow oxygen to move from the air into the venous blood and carbon dioxide to move out. The lung does other jobs too. It metabolizes some compounds, filters unwanted materials from the circulation, and acts as a reservoir for blood. But its cardinal function is to exchange gas, and we shall therefore begin at the blood-gas interface where the gas exchange occurs.

▶ Blood-Gas Interface

Oxygen and carbon dioxide move between air and blood by simple diffusion, that is, from an area of high to low partial pressure,* much as water runs downhill. Fick's law of diffusion states that the amount of gas that moves across a sheet of tissue is proportional to the area of the sheet but inversely proportional to its thickness. The blood-gas barrier is exceedingly thin (Figure 1-1) and has an area of between 50 and 100 square meters. It is therefore well suited to its function of gas exchange.

How is it possible to obtain such a prodigious surface area for diffusion inside the limited thoracic cavity? This is done by wrapping the small blood vessels (capillaries) around an enormous number of small air sacs called *alveoli* (Figure 1-2). There are about 500 million alveoli in the human lung, each about 1/3 mm in diameter. If they were spheres,[†] their total surface area would be 85 square meters, but their volume only 4 liters. By contrast, a single sphere of this volume would have an internal surface area of only 1/100 square meter. Thus, the lung generates this large diffusion area by being divided into a myriad of units.

Gas is brought to one side of the blood-gas interface by *airways*, and blood to the other side by *blood vessels*.

▶ Airways and Airflow

The airways consist of a series of branching tubes, which become narrower, shorter, and more numerous as they penetrate deeper into the lung (Figure 1-3). The *trachea* divides into right and left main bronchi, which in turn divide into lobar, then segmental bronchi. This process continues down to the *terminal bronchioles*, which are the smallest airways without alveoli. All

---

*The partial pressure of a gas is found by multiplying its concentration by the total pressure. For example, dry air has 20.93% O_2. Its partial pressure (Po_2) at sea level (barometric pressure 760 mm Hg) is 20.93/100 × 760 = 159 mm Hg. When air is inhaled into the upper airways, it is warmed and moistened, and the water vapor pressure is then 47 mm Hg, so that the total dry gas pressure is only 760 – 47 = 713 mm Hg. The Po_2 of inspired air is therefore 20.93/100 × 713 = 149 mm Hg. A liquid exposed to a gas until equilibration takes place has the same partial pressure as the gas. For a more complete description of the gas laws, see Appendix A.
[†]The alveoli are not spherical but polyhedral. Nor is the whole of their surface available for diffusion (see Figure 1-1). These numbers are therefore only approximate.

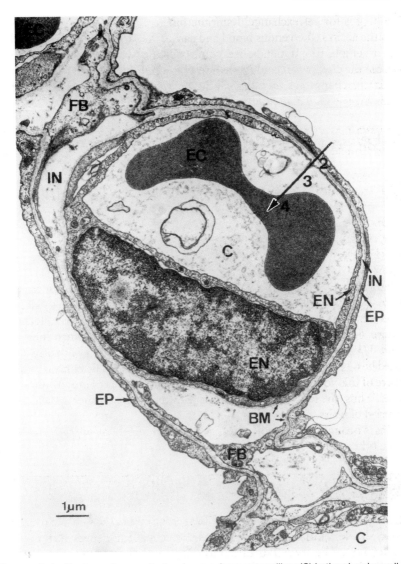

Figure 1-1. Electron micrograph showing a pulmonary capillary (C) in the alveolar wall. Note the extremely thin blood-gas barrier of about 0.3 μm in some places. The *large arrow* indicates the diffusion path from alveolar gas to the interior of the erythrocyte (EC) and includes the layer of surfactant (not shown in the preparation), alveolar epithelium (EP), interstitium (IN), capillary endothelium (EN), and plasma. Parts of structural cells called fibroblasts (FB), basement membrane (BM), and a nucleus of an endothelial cell are also seen.

of these bronchi make up the *conducting airways*. Their function is to lead inspired air to the gas-exchanging regions of the lung (Figure 1-4). Because the conducting airways contain no alveoli and therefore take no part in gas exchange, they constitute the *anatomic dead space*. Its volume is about 150 ml.

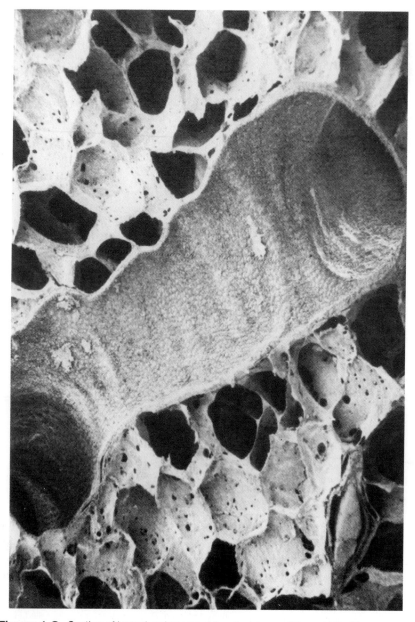

Figure 1-2. Section of lung showing many alveoli and a small bronchiole. The pulmonary capillaries run in the walls of the alveoli (Figure 1-1). The holes in the alveolar walls are the pores of Kohn.

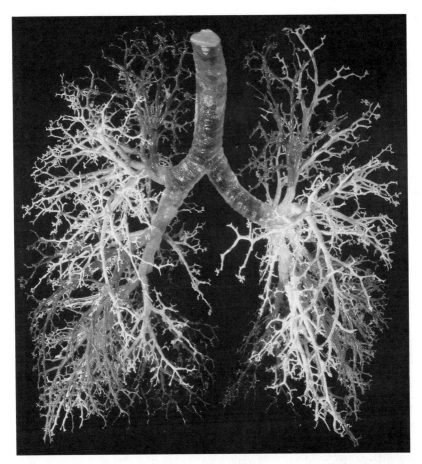

Figure 1-3. Cast of the airways of a human lung. The alveoli have been pruned away, allowing the conducting airways from the trachea to the terminal bronchioles to be seen.

The terminal bronchioles divide into *respiratory bronchioles*, which have occasional alveoli budding from their walls. Finally, we come to the *alveolar ducts*, which are completely lined with alveoli. This alveolated region of the lung where the gas exchange occurs is known as the *respiratory zone*. The portion of lung distal to a terminal bronchiole forms an anatomical unit called the *acinus*. The distance from the terminal bronchiole to the most distal alveolus is only a few millimeters, but the respiratory zone makes up most of the lung, its volume being about 2.5 to 3 liters during rest.

During inspiration, the volume of the thoracic cavity increases and air is drawn into the lung. The increase in volume is brought about partly by contraction of the diaphragm, which causes it to descend, and partly by the action of the intercostal muscles, which raise the ribs, thus increasing the cross-sectional area of the thorax. Inspired air flows down to about the terminal

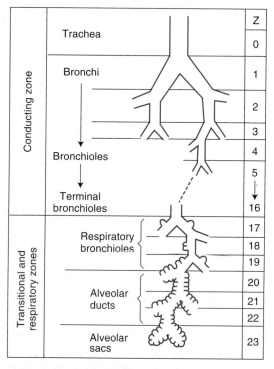

		Z
Conducting zone	Trachea	0
	Bronchi	1
		2
		3
	Bronchioles	4
		5
	Terminal bronchioles	16
Transitional and respiratory zones	Respiratory bronchioles	17
		18
		19
	Alveolar ducts	20
		21
		22
	Alveolar sacs	23

Figure 1-4. Idealization of the human airways according to Weibel. Note that the first 16 generations (Z) make up the conducting airways, and the last 7, the respiratory zone (or the transitional and respiratory zones).

bronchioles by bulk flow, like water through a hose. Beyond that point, the combined cross-sectional area of the airways is so enormous because of the large number of branches (Figure 1-5) that the forward velocity of the gas becomes small. Diffusion of gas within the airways then takes over as the dominant mechanism of ventilation in the respiratory zone. The rate of diffusion of gas molecules within the airways is so rapid and the distances to be covered so short that differences in concentration within the acinus are virtually abolished within a second. However, because the velocity of gas falls rapidly in the region of the terminal bronchioles, inhaled dust frequently settles out there.

The lung is elastic and returns passively to its preinspiratory volume during resting breathing. It is remarkably easy to distend. A normal breath of about 500 ml, for example, requires a distending pressure of less than 3 cm water. By contrast, a child's balloon may need a pressure of 30 cm water for the same change in volume.

The pressure required to move gas through the airways is also very small. During normal inspiration, an air flow rate of 1 liter. s^{-1} requires a pressure drop along the airways of less than 2 cm water. Compare a smoker's pipe, which needs a pressure of about 500 cm water for the same flow rate.

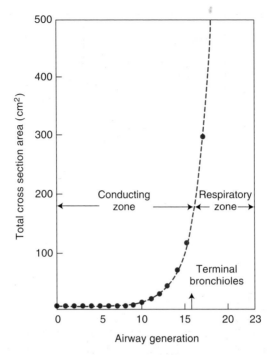

Figure 1-5. Diagram to show the extremely rapid increase in total cross-sectional area of the airways in the respiratory zone (compare Figure 1-4). As a result, the forward velocity of the gas during inspiration becomes very small in the region of the respiratory bronchioles, and gaseous diffusion becomes the chief mode of ventilation.

Airways

- Divided into a conducting zone and a respiratory zone
- Volume of the anatomic dead space is about 150 ml
- Volume of the alveolar region is about 2.5 to 3.0 liters
- Gas movement in the alveolar region is chiefly by diffusion

▶ Blood Vessels and Flow

The pulmonary blood vessels also form a series of branching tubes from the *pulmonary artery* to the *capillaries* and back to the *pulmonary veins*. Initially, the arteries, veins, and bronchi run close together, but toward the periphery of the lung, the veins move away to pass between the lobules, whereas the arteries and bronchi travel together down the centers of the lobules. The capillaries form a dense network in the walls of the alveoli

(Figure 1-6). The diameter of a capillary segment is about 7 to 10 μm, just large enough for a red blood cell. The lengths of the segments are so short that the dense network forms an almost continuous sheet of blood in the alveolar wall, a very efficient arrangement for gas exchange. Alveolar walls are not often seen face on, as in Figure 1-6. The usual, thin microscopic cross section (Figure 1-7) shows the red blood cells in the capillaries and emphasizes the enormous exposure of blood to alveolar gas, with only the thin blood-gas barrier intervening (compare Figure 1-1).

The extreme thinness of the blood-gas barrier means that the capillaries are easily damaged. Increasing the pressure in the capillaries to high levels or inflating the lung to high volumes, for example, can raise the wall stresses of the capillaries to the point at which ultrastructural changes can occur. The capillaries then leak plasma and even red blood cells into the alveolar spaces.

The pulmonary artery receives the whole output of the right heart, but the resistance of the pulmonary circuit is astonishingly small. A mean pulmonary arterial pressure of only about 20 cm water (about 15 mm Hg) is required for a flow of 6 liter·min^{-1} (the same flow through a soda straw needs 120 cm water).

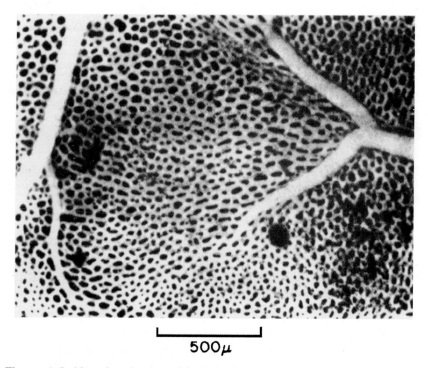

500μ

Figure 1-6. View of an alveolar wall (in the frog) showing the dense network of capillaries. A small artery (*left*) and vein (*right*) can also be seen. The individual capillary segments are so short that the blood forms an almost continuous sheet.

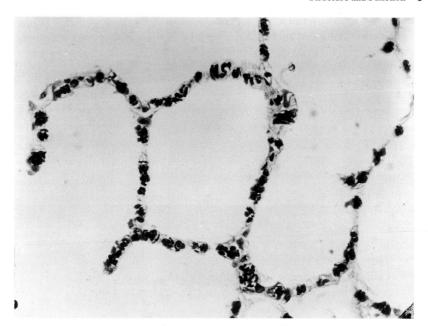

Figure 1-7. Microscopic section of dog lung showing capillaries in the alveolar walls. The blood-gas barrier is so thin that it cannot be identified here (compare Figure 1-1). This section was prepared from lung that was rapidly frozen while being perfused.

Each red blood cell spends about 0.75 second in the capillary network and during this time probably traverses two or three alveoli. So efficient is the anatomy for gas exchange that this brief time is sufficient for virtually complete equilibration of oxygen and carbon dioxide between alveolar gas and capillary blood.

The lung has an additional blood system, the bronchial circulation that supplies the conducting airways down to about the terminal bronchioles. Some of this blood is carried away from the lung via the pulmonary veins, and some enters the systemic circulation. The flow through the bronchial circulation is a mere fraction of that through the pulmonary circulation, and the lung can function fairly well without it, for example, following lung transplantation.

Blood-Gas Interface

- Extremely thin (0.2–0.3 μm) over much of its area
- Enormous surface area of 50 to 100 m²
- Large area obtained by having about 500 million alveoli
- So thin that large increases in capillary pressure can damage the barrier

To conclude this brief account of the functional anatomy of the lung, let us glance at two special problems that the lung has overcome.

▶ Stability of Alveoli

The lung can be regarded as a collection of 500 million bubbles, each 0.3 mm in diameter. Such a structure is inherently unstable. Because of the surface tension of the liquid lining the alveoli, relatively large forces develop that tend to collapse alveoli. Fortunately, some of the cells lining the alveoli secrete a material called *surfactant* that dramatically lowers the surface tension of the alveolar lining layer (see Chapter 7). As a consequence, the stability of the alveoli is enormously increased, although collapse of small air spaces is always a potential problem and frequently occurs in disease.

Blood Vessels

- The whole of the output of the right heart goes to the lung
- The diameter of the capillaries is about 7 to 10 μm
- The thickness of much of the capillary walls is less than 0.3 μm
- Blood spends about 0.75 second in the capillaries

▶ Removal of Inhaled Particles

With its surface area of 50 to 100 square meters, the lung presents the largest surface of the body to an increasingly hostile environment. Various mechanisms for dealing with inhaled particles have been developed (see Chapter 9). Large particles are filtered out in the nose. Smaller particles that deposit in the conducting airways are removed by a moving staircase of mucus that continually sweeps debris up to the epiglottis, where it is swallowed. The mucus, secreted by mucous glands and also by goblet cells in the bronchial walls, is propelled by millions of tiny cilia, which move rhythmically under normal conditions but are paralyzed by some inhaled toxins.

The alveoli have no cilia, and particles that deposit there are engulfed by large wandering cells called macrophages. The foreign material is then removed from the lung via the lymphatics or the blood flow. Blood cells such as leukocytes also participate in the defense reaction to foreign material.

KEY CONCEPTS

1. The blood-gas barrier is extremely thin with a very large area, making it ideal for gas exchange by passive diffusion.
2. The conducting airways extend to the terminal bronchioles, with a total volume of about 150 ml. All the gas exchange occurs in the respiratory zone, which has a volume of about 2.5 to 3 liters.

3. Convective flow takes inspired gas to about the terminal bronchioles; beyond this, gas movement is increasingly by diffusion in the alveolar region.
4. The pulmonary capillaries occupy a huge area of the alveolar wall, and a red cell spends about 0.75 second in them.

QUESTIONS

For each question, choose the one best answer.

1. Concerning the blood-gas barrier of the human lung,
   A. The thinnest part of the blood-gas barrier has a thickness of about 3 μm.
   B. The total area of the blood-gas barrier is about 1 square meter.
   C. About 10% of the area of the alveolar wall is occupied by capillaries.
   D. If the pressure in the capillaries rises to unphysiologically high levels, the blood-gas barrier can be damaged.
   E. Oxygen crosses the blood-gas barrier by active transport.

2. When oxygen moves through the thin side of the blood-gas barrier from the alveolar gas to the hemoglobin of the red blood cell, it traverses the following layers in order:
   A. Epithelial cell, surfactant, interstitium, endothelial cell, plasma, red cell membrane.
   B. Surfactant, epithelial cell, interstitium, endothelial cell, plasma, red cell membrane.
   C. Surfactant, endothelial cell, interstitium, epithelial cell, plasma, red cell membrane.
   D. Epithelium cell, interstitium, endothelial cell, plasma, red cell membrane.
   E. Surfactant, epithelial cell, interstitium, endothelial cell, red cell membrane.

3. What is the P_{O_2} (in mm Hg) of moist inspired gas of a climber on the summit of Mt. Everest (assume barometric pressure is 247 mm Hg)?
   A. 32
   B. 42
   C. 52
   D. 62
   E. 72

4. Concerning the airways of the human lung,
   A. The volume of the conducting zone is about 50 ml.
   B. The volume of the rest of the lung during resting conditions is about 5 liters.
   C. A respiratory bronchiole can be distinguished from a terminal bronchiole because the latter has alveoli in its walls.
   D. On the average, there are about three branchings of the conducting airways before the first alveoli appear in their walls.
   E. In the alveolar ducts, the predominant mode of gas flow is diffusion rather than convection.

5. Concerning the blood vessels of the human lung,
   A. The pulmonary veins form a branching pattern that matches that of the airways.
   B. The average diameter of the capillaries is about 50 μm.
   C. The bronchial circulation has about the same blood flow as the pulmonary circulation.
   D. On the average, blood spends about 0.75 second in the capillaries under resting conditions.
   E. The mean pressure in the pulmonary artery is about 100 mm Hg.

Ventilation

2

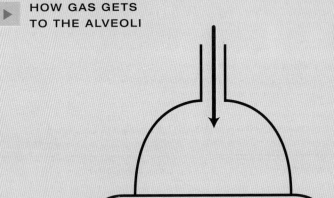

We now look in more detail at how oxygen is brought to the blood-gas barrier by the process of ventilation. First, lung volumes are briefly reviewed. Then total ventilation and alveolar ventilation, which is the amount of fresh gas getting to the alveoli, are discussed. The lung that does not participate in gas exchange is dealt with under the headings of anatomic and physiologic dead space. Finally, the uneven distribution of ventilation caused by gravity is introduced.

► Lung Volumes
► Ventilation
► Anatomic Dead Space
► Physiologic Dead Space
► Regional Differences in Ventilation

The next three chapters concern how inspired air gets to the alveoli, how gases cross the blood-gas interface, and how they are removed from the lung by the blood. These functions are carried out by ventilation, diffusion, and blood flow, respectively.

Figure 2-1 is a highly simplified diagram of a lung. The various bronchi that make up the conducting airways (Figures 1-3 and 1-4) are now represented by a single tube labeled "anatomic dead space." This leads into the gas-exchanging region of the lung, which is bounded by the blood-gas interface and the pulmonary capillary blood. With each inspiration, about 500 ml of air enters the lung (*tidal volume*). Note how small a proportion of the total lung volume is represented by the anatomic dead space. Also note the very small volume of capillary blood compared with that of alveolar gas (compare Figure 1-7).

▶ Lung Volumes

Before looking at the movement of gas into the lung, a brief glance at the static volumes of the lung is helpful. Some of these can be measured with a spirometer (Figure 2-2). During exhalation, the bell goes up and the pen down, marking a moving chart. First, normal breathing can be seen (*tidal volume*). Next, the subject took a maximal inspiration and followed this by a maximal expiration. The exhaled volume is called the *vital capacity*. However, some gas remained in the lung after a maximal expiration; this is the *residual volume*. The volume of gas in the lung after a normal expiration is the *functional residual capacity (FRC)*.

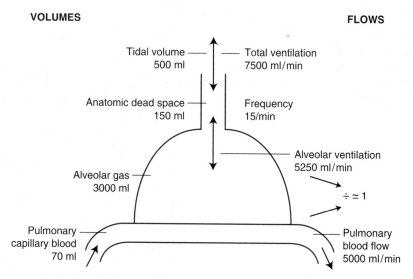

Figure 2-1. Diagram of a lung showing typical volumes and flows. There is considerable variation around these values.

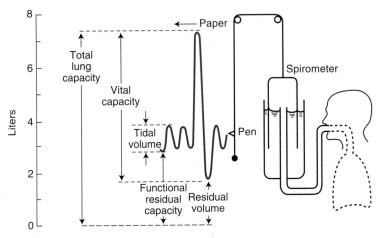

Figure 2-2. Lung volumes. Note that the total lung capacity, functional residual capacity, and residual volume cannot be measured with the spirometer.

Neither the FRC nor the residual volume can be measured with a simple spirometer. However, a gas dilution technique can be used, as shown in Figure 2-3. The subject is connected to a spirometer containing a known concentration of helium, which is virtually insoluble in blood. After some breaths, the helium concentrations in the spirometer and lung become the same.

Because no helium has been lost, the amount of helium present before equilibration (concentration times volume) is

$$C_1 \times V_1$$

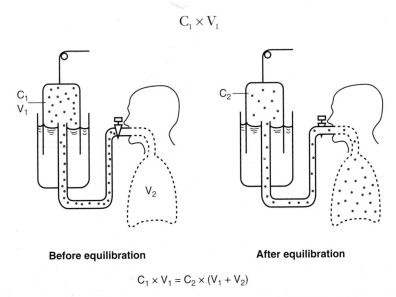

$$C_1 \times V_1 = C_2 \times (V_1 + V_2)$$

Figure 2-3. Measurement of the functional residual capacity by helium dilution.

and equals the amount after equilibration:

$$C_2 \times (V_1 + V_2)$$

From this,

$$V_2 = V_1 \times \frac{C_1 - C_2}{C_2}$$

In practice, oxygen is added to the spirometer during equilibration to make up for that consumed by the subject, and also carbon dioxide is absorbed.

Another way of measuring the FRC is with a body plethysmograph (Figure 2-4). This is a large airtight box, like an old telephone booth, in which the subject sits. At the end of a normal expiration, a shutter closes the mouthpiece and the subject is asked to make respiratory efforts. As the subject tries to inhale, he (or she) expands the gas in his lungs; lung volume increases, and the box pressure rises because its gas volume decreases. Boyle's law states that pressure × volume is constant (at constant temperature).

Therefore, if the pressures in the box before and after the inspiratory effort are P_1 and P_2, respectively, V_1 is the preinspiratory box volume, and ΔV is the change in volume of the box (or lung), we can write

$$P_1 V_1 = P_2 (V_1 - \Delta V)$$

Thus, ΔV can be obtained.

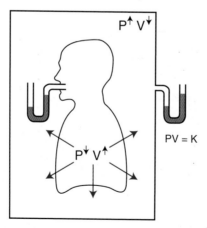

Figure 2-4. Measurement of FRC with a body plethysmograph. When the subject makes an inspiratory effort against a closed airway, he slightly increases the volume of his lung, airway pressure decreases, and box pressure increases. From Boyle's law, lung volume is obtained (see text).

Next, Boyle's law is applied to the gas in the lung. Now,

$$P_3V_2 = P_4(V_2 + \Delta V)$$

where P_3 and P_4 are the mouth pressures before and after the inspiratory effort, and V_2 is the FRC. Thus, FRC can be obtained.

The body plethysmograph measures the total volume of gas in the lung, including any that is trapped behind closed airways (an example is shown in Figure 7-9) and that therefore does not communicate with the mouth. By contrast, the helium dilution method measures only communicating gas or ventilated lung volume. In young normal subjects, these volumes are virtually the same, but in patients with lung disease, the ventilated volume may be considerably less than the total volume because of gas trapped behind obstructed airways.

Lung Volumes

- Tidal volume and vital capacity can be measured with a simple spirometer
- Total lung capacity, functional residual capacity, and residual volume need an additional measurement by helium dilution or the body plethysmograph
- Helium is used because of its very low solubility in blood
- The use of the body plethysmograph depends on Boyle's law, PV = K, at constant temperature

---

▶ Ventilation

Suppose the volume exhaled with each breath is 500 ml (Figure 2-1) and there are 15 breaths·min⁻¹. Then the total volume leaving the lung each minute is $500 \times 15 = 7500$ ml·min⁻¹. This is known as the *total ventilation*. The volume of air entering the lung is very slightly greater because more oxygen is taken in than carbon dioxide is given out.

However, not all the air that passes the lips reaches the alveolar gas compartment where gas exchange occurs. Of each 500 ml inhaled in Figure 2-1, 150 ml remains behind in the anatomic dead space. Thus, the volume of fresh gas entering the respiratory zone each minute is $(500 - 150) \times 15$ or 5250 ml·min⁻¹. This is called the *alveolar ventilation* and is of key importance because it represents the amount of fresh inspired air available for gas exchange (strictly, the alveolar ventilation is also measured on expiration, but the volume is almost the same).

The total ventilation can be measured easily by having the subject breathe through a valve box that separates the inspired from the expired gas, and

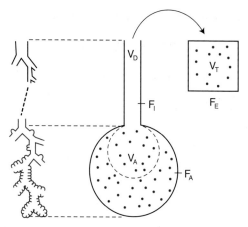

Figure 2-5. The tidal volume (V_T) is a mixture of gas from the anatomic dead space (V_D) and a contribution from the alveolar gas (V_A). The concentrations of CO_2 are shown by the *dots*. F, fractional concentration; I, inspired; E, expired. Compare Figure 1-4.

collecting all the expired gas in a bag. The alveolar ventilation is more difficult to determine. One way is to measure the volume of the anatomic dead space (see below) and calculate the dead space ventilation (volume × respiratory frequency). This is then subtracted from the total ventilation.

We can summarize this conveniently with symbols (Figure 2-5). Using V to denote volume, and the subscripts T, D, and A to denote tidal, dead space, and alveolar, respectively,

$$V_T = V_D + V_A{}^*$$

therefore,

$$V_T \cdot n = V_D \cdot n + V_A \cdot n$$

where n is the respiratory frequency.

Therefore,

$$\dot{V}_E = \dot{V}_D - \dot{V}_A$$

where $\dot{V}$ means volume per unit time, $\dot{V}_E$ is expired total ventilation, and $\dot{V}_D$ and $\dot{V}_A$ are the dead space and alveolar ventilations, respectively (see Appendix A for a summary of symbols).

Thus,

$$\dot{V}_A = \dot{V}_E - \dot{V}_D$$

---

*Note that V_A here means the volume of alveolar gas in the tidal volume, not the total volume of alveolar gas in the lung.

A difficulty with this method is that the anatomic dead space is not easy to measure, although a value for it can be assumed with little error. Note that alveolar ventilation can be increased by raising either tidal volume or respiratory frequency (or both). Increasing tidal volume is often more effective because this reduces the proportion of each breath occupied by the anatomic dead space.

Another way of measuring alveolar ventilation in normal subjects is from the concentration of CO_2 in expired gas (Figure 2-5). Because no gas exchange occurs in the anatomic dead space, there is no CO_2 there at the end of inspiration (we can neglect the small amount of CO_2 in the air). Thus, because all the expired CO_2 comes from the alveolar gas,

$$\dot{V}_{CO_2} = \dot{V}_A \times \frac{\%CO_2}{100}$$

The $\%CO_2/100$ is often called the fractional concentration and is denoted by F_{CO_2}.

Therefore,

$$\dot{V}_{CO_2} = \dot{V}_A \times F_{CO_2}$$

and rearranging gives

$$\dot{V}_A = \frac{\dot{V}_{CO_2}}{F_{CO_2}}$$

Thus, the alveolar ventilation can be obtained by dividing the CO_2 output by the alveolar fractional concentration of this **gas.**

Note that the partial pressure of CO_2 (denoted P_{CO_2}) is proportional to the fractional concentration of the gas in the alveoli, or $P_{CO_2} = F_{CO_2} \times K$, where K is a constant.

Therefore,

$$\dot{V}_A = \frac{\dot{V}_{CO_2}}{P_{CO_2}} \times K$$

This is called the alveolar ventilation equation.

Because in normal subjects the P_{CO_2} of alveolar gas and arterial blood are virtually identical, the arterial P_{CO_2} can be used to determine alveolar ventilation. The relation between alveolar ventilation and P_{CO_2} is of crucial importance. If the alveolar ventilation is halved (and CO_2 production remains unchanged), for example, the alveolar and arterial P_{CO_2} will double.

▶ Anatomic Dead Space

This is the volume of the conducting airways (Figures 1-3 and 1-4). The normal value is about 150 ml, and it increases with large inspirations because of the traction or pull exerted on the bronchi by the surrounding lung parenchyma. The dead space also depends on the size and posture of the subject.

The volume of the anatomic dead space can be measured by *Fowler's method*. The subject breathes through a valve box, and the sampling tube of a rapid nitrogen analyzer continuously samples gas at the lips (Figure 2-6A). Following a single inspiration of 100% O_2, the N_2 concentration rises as the dead space gas is increasingly washed out by alveolar gas. Finally, an almost uniform gas concentration is seen, representing pure alveolar gas. This phase is often called the alveolar "plateau," although in normal subjects it is not quite flat, and in patients with lung disease it may rise steeply. Expired volume is also recorded.

The dead space is found by plotting N_2 concentration against expired volume and drawing a vertical line such that area A is equal to area B in Figure 2-6B. The dead space is the volume expired up to the vertical line. In effect, this method measures the volume of the conducting airways down to the midpoint of the transition from dead space to alveolar gas.

▶ Physiologic Dead Space

Another way of measuring dead space is *Bohr's method*. Figure 2-5 shows that all the expired CO_2 comes from the alveolar gas and none from the dead space. Therefore, we can write

$$V_T \cdot F_E = V_A \cdot F_A$$

Now,

$$V_T = V_A + V_D$$

Therefore,

$$V_A = V_T - V_D$$

substituting

$$V_T \cdot F_E = (V_T - V_D) \cdot F_A$$

whence

$$\frac{V_D}{V_T} = \frac{P_{A_{CO_2}} - P_{E_{CO_2}}}{P_{A_{CO_2}}} \quad \text{(Bohr equation)}$$

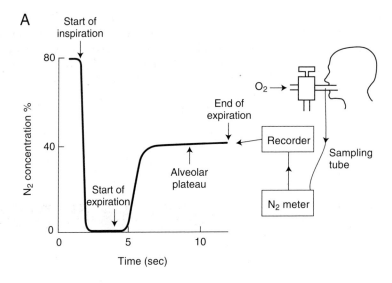

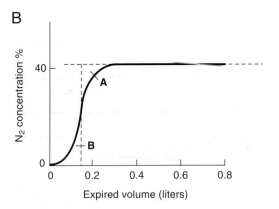

Figure 2-6. Fowler's method of measuring the anatomic dead space with a rapid N_2 analyzer. **A** shows that following a test inspiration of 100% O_2, the N_2 concentration rises during expiration to an almost level "plateau" representing pure alveolar gas. In **(B)**, N_2 concentration is plotted against expired volume, and the dead space is the volume up to the *vertical dashed line*, which makes the areas A and B equal.

where A and E refer to alveolar and mixed expired, respectively (see Appendix A). The normal ratio of dead space to tidal volume is in the range of 0.2 to 0.35 during resting breathing. In normal subjects, the P_{CO_2} in alveolar gas and that in arterial blood are virtually identical so that the equation is therefore often written

$$\frac{V_D}{V_T} = \frac{P_{A_{CO_2}} - P_{E_{CO_2}}}{P_{A_{CO_2}}}$$

It should be noted that Fowler's and Bohr's methods measure somewhat different things. Fowler's method measures the volume of the conducting airways down to the level where the rapid dilution of inspired gas occurs with gas already in the lung. This volume is determined by the geometry of the rapidly expanding airways (Figure 1-5), and because it reflects the morphology of the lung, it is called the *anatomic dead space*. Bohr's method measures the volume of the lung that does not eliminate CO_2. Because this is a functional measurement, the volume is called the *physiologic dead space*. In normal subjects, the volumes are very nearly the same. However, in patients with lung disease, the physiologic dead space may be considerably larger because of inequality of blood flow and ventilation within the lung (see Chapter 5).

Ventilation

- Total ventilation is tidal volume × respiratory frequency
- Alveolar ventilation is the amount of fresh gas getting to the alveoli, or $(V_T - V_D) \times n$
- Anatomic dead space is the volume of the conducting airways, about 150 ml
- Physiologic dead space is the volume of gas that does not eliminate CO_2
- The two dead spaces are almost the same in normal subjects, but the physiologic dead space is increased in many lung diseases

---

► Regional Differences in Ventilation

So far, we have been assuming that all regions of the normal lung have the same ventilation. However, it has been shown that the lower regions of the lung ventilate better than do the upper zones. This can be demonstrated if a subject inhales radioactive xenon gas (Figure 2-7). When the xenon-133 enters the counting field, its radiation penetrates the chest wall and can be recorded by a bank of counters or a radiation camera. In this way, the volume of the inhaled xenon going to various regions can be determined.

Figure 2-7 shows the results obtained in a series of normal volunteers using this method. It can be seen that ventilation per unit volume is greatest near the bottom of the lung and becomes progressively smaller toward the top. Other measurements show that when the subject is in the supine position, this difference disappears, with the result that apical and basal ventilations become the same. However, in that posture, the ventilation of the lowermost (posterior) lung exceeds that of the uppermost (anterior) lung. Again, in the lateral position (subject on his side), the dependent lung is best ventilated. The cause of these regional differences in ventilation is dealt with in Chapter 7.

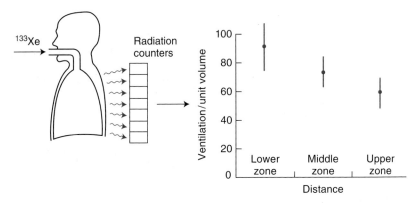

Figure 2-7. Measurement of regional differences in ventilation with radioactive xenon. When the gas is inhaled, its radiation can be detected by counters outside the chest. Note that the ventilation decreases from the lower to upper regions of the upright lung.

KEY CONCEPTS

1. Lung volumes that cannot be measured with a simple spirometer include the total lung capacity, the functional residual capacity, and the residual volume. These can be determined by helium dilution or the body plethysmograph.
2. Alveolar ventilation is the volume of fresh (non–dead space) gas entering the respiratory zone per minute. It can be determined from the alveolar ventilation equation, that is, the CO_2 output divided by the fractional concentration of CO_2 in the expired gas.
3. The concentration of CO_2 (and therefore its partial pressure) in alveolar gas and arterial blood is inversely related to the alveolar ventilation.
4. The anatomic dead space is the volume of the conducting airways and can be measured from the nitrogen concentration following a single inspiration of oxygen.
5. The physiologic dead space is the volume of lung that does not eliminate CO_2. It is measured by Bohr's method using arterial and expired CO_2.
6. The lower regions of the lung are better ventilated than the upper regions because of the effects of gravity on the lung.

Questions

For each question, choose the one best answer.

1. The only variable in the following list that cannot be measured with a simple spirometer and stopwatch is
   A. Tidal volume.
   B. Functional residual capacity.
   C. Vital capacity.
   D. Total ventilation.
   E. Respiratory frequency.

2. Concerning the pulmonary acinus,

    A. Less than 90% oxygen uptake of the lung occurs in the acini.

    B. Percentage change in volume of the acini during inspiration is less than that of the whole lung.

    C. Volume of the acini is less than 90% of the total volume of the lung at FRC.

    D. Each acinus is supplied by a terminal bronchiole.

    E. The ventilation of the acini at the base of the upright human lung at FRC is less than those at the apex.

3. In a measurement of FRC by helium dilution, the original and final helium concentrations were 10% and 6%, and the spirometer volume was kept at 5 liters. What was the volume of the FRC in liters?

    A. 2.5
    B. 3.0
    C. 3.3
    D. 3.8
    E. 5.0

4. A patient sits in a body plethysmograph (body box) and makes an expiratory effort against his closed glottis. What happens to the following: pressure in the lung airways, lung volume, box pressure, box volume?

	Airway Pressure	Lung Volume	Box Pressure	Box Volume
A.	↓	↑	↑	↓
B.	↓	↑	↓	↑
C.	↑	↓	↑	↓
D.	↑	↓	↓	↑
E.	↑	↑	↓	↓

5. If CO_2 production remains constant and alveolar ventilation is increased threefold, the alveolar P_{CO_2} after a steady state is reached will be what percentage of its former value?

    A. 25
    B. 33
    C. 50
    D. 100
    E. 300

6. In a measurement of physiologic dead space using Bohr's method, the alveolar and mixed expired P_{CO_2} were 40 and 30 mm Hg, respectively. What was the ratio of dead space to tidal volume?

    A. 0.20
    B. 0.25
    C. 0.30
    D. 0.35
    E. 0.40

Diffusion

3

We now consider how gases move across the blood-gas barrier by diffusion. First, the basic laws of diffusion are introduced. Next, we distinguish between diffusion- and perfusion-limited gases. Oxygen uptake along the pulmonary capillary is then analyzed, and there is a section on the measurement of diffusing capacity using carbon monoxide. The finite reaction rate of oxygen with hemoglobin is conveniently considered with diffusion. Finally, there is a brief reference to the interpretation of measurements of diffusing capacity and possible limitations of carbon dioxide diffusion.

In the last chapter, we looked at how gas is moved from the atmosphere to the alveoli, or in the reverse direction. We now come to the transfer of gas across the blood-gas barrier. This process occurs by *diffusion*. Only 70 years ago, some physiologists believed that the lung secreted oxygen into the capillaries, that is, the oxygen was moved from a region of lower to one of higher partial pressure. Such a process was thought to occur in the swim bladder of fish, and it requires energy. But more accurate measurements showed that this does not occur in the lung and that all gases move across the alveolar wall by passive diffusion.

▶ Laws of Diffusion

Diffusion through tissues is described by Fick's law (Figure 3-1). This states that the rate of transfer of a gas through a sheet of tissue is proportional to the tissue area and the difference in gas partial pressure between the two sides, and inversely proportional to the tissue thickness. As we have seen, the area of the blood-gas barrier in the lung is enormous (50 to 100 square meters), and the thickness is only 0.3 μm in many places (Figure 1-1), so the dimensions of the barrier are ideal for diffusion. In addition, the rate of transfer is proportional to a diffusion constant, which depends on the properties of the tissue and the particular gas. The constant is proportional to the solubility of the gas and inversely proportional to the square root of the molecular weight (Figure 3-1). This means that CO_2 diffuses about 20 times more rapidly than does O_2 through tissue sheets because it has a much higher solubility but not a very different molecular weight.

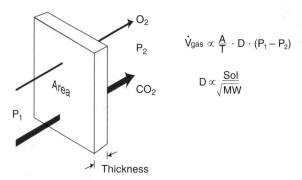

$$\dot{V}_{gas} \propto \frac{A}{T} \cdot D \cdot (P_1 - P_2)$$

$$D \propto \frac{Sol}{\sqrt{MW}}$$

Figure 3-1. Diffusion through a tissue sheet. The amount of gas transferred is proportional to the area (A), a diffusion constant (D), and the difference in partial pressure $(P_1 - P_2)$, and is inversely proportional to the thickness (T). The constant is proportional to the gas solubility (Sol) but inversely proportional to the square root of its molecular weight (MW).

Fick's Law of Diffusion

- The rate of diffusion of a gas through a tissue slice is proportional to the area but inversely proportional to the thickness
- Diffusion rate is proportional to the partial pressure difference
- Diffusion rate is proportional to the solubility of the gas in the tissue but inversely proportional to the square root of the molecular weight

► Diffusion and Perfusion Limitations

Suppose a red blood cell enters a pulmonary capillary of an alveolus that contains a foreign gas such as carbon monoxide or nitrous oxide. How rapidly will the partial pressure in the blood rise? Figure 3-2 shows the time courses as the red blood cell moves through the capillary, a process that takes about 0.75 second. Look first at carbon monoxide. When the red cell enters the

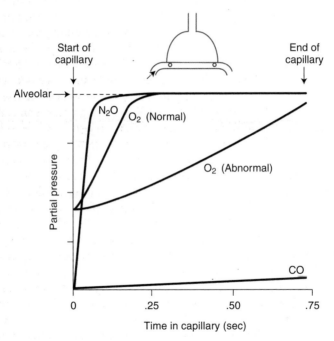

Figure 3-2. Uptake of carbon monoxide, nitrous oxide, and O_2 along the pulmonary capillary. Note that the blood partial pressure of nitrous oxide virtually reaches that of alveolar gas very early in the capillary, so the transfer of this gas is perfusion limited. By contrast, the partial pressure of carbon monoxide in the blood is almost unchanged, so its transfer is diffusion limited. O_2 transfer can be perfusion limited or partly diffusion limited, depending on the conditions.

capillary, carbon monoxide moves rapidly across the extremely thin blood-gas barrier from the alveolar gas into the cell. As a result, the content of carbon monoxide in the cell rises. However, because of the tight bond that forms between carbon monoxide and hemoglobin within the cell, a large amount of carbon monoxide can be taken up by the cell with almost no increase in partial pressure. Thus, as the cell moves through the capillary, the carbon monoxide partial pressure in the blood hardly changes, so that no appreciable back pressure develops, and the gas continues to move rapidly across the alveolar wall. It is clear, therefore, that the amount of carbon monoxide that gets into the blood is limited by the diffusion properties of the blood-gas barrier and not by the amount of blood available.* The transfer of carbon monoxide is therefore said to be *diffusion limited*.

Contrast the time course of nitrous oxide. When this gas moves across the alveolar wall into the blood, no combination with hemoglobin takes place. As a result, the blood has nothing like the avidity for nitrous oxide that it has for carbon monoxide, and the partial pressure rises rapidly. Indeed, Figure 3-2 shows that the partial pressure of nitrous oxide in the blood has virtually reached that of the alveolar gas by the time the red cell is only one-tenth of the way along the capillary. After this point, almost no nitrous oxide is transferred. Thus, the amount of this gas taken up by the blood depends entirely on the amount of available blood flow and not at all on the diffusion properties of the blood-gas barrier. The transfer of nitrous oxide is therefore *perfusion limited*.

What of O_2? Its time course lies between those of carbon monoxide and nitrous oxide. O_2 combines with hemoglobin (unlike nitrous oxide) but with nothing like the avidity of carbon monoxide. In other words, the rise in partial pressure when O_2 enters a red blood cell is much greater than is the case for the same number of molecules of carbon monoxide. Figure 3-2 shows that the Po_2 of the red blood cell as it enters the capillary is already about four-tenths of the alveolar value because of the O_2 in mixed venous blood. Under typical resting conditions, the capillary Po_2 virtually reaches that of alveolar gas when the red cell is about one-third of the way along the capillary. Under these conditions, O_2 transfer is perfusion limited like nitrous oxide. However, in some abnormal circumstances when the diffusion properties of the lung are impaired, for example, because of thickening of the blood-gas barrier, the blood Po_2 does not reach the alveolar value by the end of the capillary, and now there is some diffusion limitation as well.

A more detailed analysis shows that whether a gas is diffusion limited or not depends essentially on its solubility in the blood-gas barrier compared with its "solubility" in blood (actually the slope of the dissociation curve; see Chapter 6). For a gas like carbon monoxide, these are very different, whereas for a gas like nitrous oxide, they are the same. An analogy is the rate at which sheep can enter a field through a gate. If the gate is narrow but the field is

---

*This introductory description of carbon monoxide transfer is not completely accurate because of the rate of reaction of carbon monoxide with hemoglobin (see later).

large, the number of sheep that can enter in a given time is limited by the size of the gate. However, if both the gate and the field are small (or both are big), the number of sheep is limited by the size of the field.

▶ Oxygen Uptake Along the Pulmonary Capillary

Let us take a closer look at the uptake of O_2 by blood as it moves through a pulmonary capillary. Figure 3-3A shows that the Po_2 in a red blood cell entering the capillary is normally about 40 mm Hg. Across the blood-gas barrier, only 0.3 μm away, is the alveolar Po_2 of 100 mm Hg. Oxygen floods down

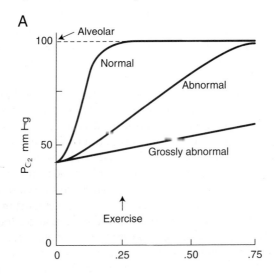

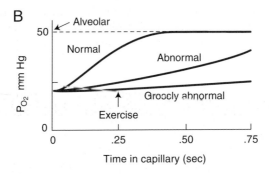

Time in capillary (sec)

Figure 3-3. Oxygen time courses in the pulmonary capillary when diffusion is normal and abnormal (e.g., because of thickening of the blood-gas barrier by disease). **A** shows time courses when the alveolar Po_2 is normal. **B** shows slower oxygenation when the alveolar Po_2 is abnormally low. Note that in both cases, severe exercise reduces the time available for oxygenation.

this large pressure gradient, and the P_{O_2} in the red cell rapidly rises; indeed, as we have seen, it very nearly reaches the P_{O_2} of alveolar gas by the time the red cell is only one-third of its way along the capillary. Thus, under normal circumstances, the difference in P_{O_2} between alveolar gas and end-capillary blood is immeasurably small—a mere fraction of an mm Hg. In other words, the diffusion reserves of the normal lung are enormous.

With severe exercise, the pulmonary blood flow is greatly increased, and the time normally spent by the red cell in the capillary, about 0.75 second, may be reduced to as little as one-third of this. Therefore, the time available for oxygenation is less, but in normal subjects breathing air, there is generally still no measurable fall in end-capillary P_{O_2}. However, if the blood-gas barrier is markedly thickened by disease so that oxygen diffusion is impeded, the rate of rise of P_{O_2} in the red blood cells is correspondingly slow, and the P_{O_2} may not reach that of alveolar gas before the time available for oxygenation in the capillary has run out. In this case, a measurable difference between alveolar gas and end-capillary blood for P_{O_2} may occur.

Another way of stressing the diffusion properties of the lung is to lower the alveolar P_{O_2} (Figure 3-3B). Suppose that this has been reduced to 50 mm Hg, by the subject either going to high altitude or inhaling a low O_2 mixture. Now, although the P_{O_2} in the red cell at the start of the capillary may only be about 20 mm Hg, the partial pressure difference responsible for driving the O_2 across the blood-gas barrier has been reduced from 60 mm Hg (Figure 3-3A) to only 30 mm Hg. O_2 therefore moves across more slowly. In addition, the rate of rise of P_{O_2} for a given increase in O_2 concentration in the blood is less than it was because of the steep slope of the O_2 dissociation curve when the P_{O_2} is low (see Chapter 6). For both of these reasons, therefore, the rise in P_{O_2} along the capillary is relatively slow, and failure to reach the alveolar P_{O_2} is more likely. Thus, severe exercise at very high altitude is one of the few situations in which diffusion impairment of O_2 transfer in normal subjects can be convincingly demonstrated. By the same token, patients with a thickened blood-gas barrier will be most likely to show evidence of diffusion impairment if they breathe a low oxygen mixture, especially if they exercise as well.

Diffusion of Oxygen Across the Blood-Gas Barrier

- At rest, the P_{O_2} of the blood virtually reaches that of the alveolar gas after about one-third of its time in the capillary
- Blood spends only about 0.75 second in the capillary at rest
- On exercise, the time is reduced to perhaps 0.25 second
- The diffusion process is challenged by exercise, alveolar hypoxia, and thickening of the blood-gas barrier

▶ Measurement of Diffusing Capacity

We have seen that oxygen transfer into the pulmonary capillary is normally limited by the amount of blood flow available, although under some circumstances diffusion limitation also occurs (Figure 3-2). By contrast, the transfer of carbon monoxide is limited solely by diffusion, and it is therefore the gas of choice for measuring the diffusion properties of the lung. At one time O_2 was employed under hypoxic conditions (Figure 3-3B), but this technique is no longer used.

The laws of diffusion (Figure 3-1) state that the amount of gas transferred across a sheet of tissue is proportional to the area, a diffusion constant, and the difference in partial pressure, and inversely proportional to the thickness, or

$$\dot{V}_{gas} = \frac{A}{T} \cdot D \cdot (P_1 - P_2)$$

Now, for a complex structure like the blood-gas barrier of the lung, it is not possible to measure the area and thickness during life. Instead, the equation is rewritten

$$V_{gas} = D_L \cdot (P_1 - P_2)$$

where D_L is called the *diffusing capacity of the lung* and includes the area, thickness, and diffusion properties of the sheet and the gas concerned. Thus, the diffusing capacity for carbon monoxide is given by

$$D_L = \frac{\dot{V}_{CO}}{P_1 - P_2}$$

where P_1 and P_2 are the partial pressures of alveolar gas and capillary blood, respectively. But as we have seen (Figure 3-2), the partial pressure of carbon monoxide in capillary blood is extremely small and can generally be neglected. Thus,

$$D_L = \frac{\dot{V}_{CO}}{P_{A_{CO}}}$$

or, in words, the diffusing capacity of the lung for carbon monoxide is the volume of carbon monoxide transferred in milliliters per minute per mm Hg of alveolar partial pressure.

Measurement of Diffusing Capacity

- Carbon monoxide is used because the uptake of this gas is diffusion limited
- Normal diffusing capacity is about 25 ml·min^{-1}·mm Hg^{-1}
- Diffusing capacity increases on exercise

A frequently used test is the *single-breath method*, in which a single inspiration of a dilute mixture of carbon monoxide is made and the rate of disappearance of carbon monoxide from the alveolar gas during a 10-second breathhold is calculated. This is usually done by measuring the inspired and expired concentrations of carbon monoxide with an infrared analyzer. The alveolar concentration of carbon monoxide is not constant during the breath-holding period, but allowance can be made for that. Helium is also added to the inspired gas to give a measurement of lung volume by dilution.

The normal value of the diffusing capacity for carbon monoxide at rest is about 25 ml·min^{-1}·mm Hg^{-1}, and it increases to two or three times this value on exercise because of recruitment and distension of pulmonary capillaries (see Chapter 4).

▶ Reaction Rates with Hemoglobin

So far we have assumed that all the resistance to the movement of O_2 and CO resides in the barrier between blood and gas. However, Figure 1-1 shows that the path length from the alveolar wall to the center of a red blood cell exceeds that in the wall itself, so that some of the diffusion resistance is located within the capillary. In addition, there is another type of resistance to gas transfer that is most conveniently discussed with diffusion, that is, the resistance caused by the finite rate of reaction of O_2 or CO with hemoglobin inside the red blood cell.

When O_2 (or CO) is added to blood, its combination with hemoglobin is quite fast, being well on the way to completion in 0.2 second. However, oxygenation occurs so rapidly in the pulmonary capillary (Figure 3-3) that even this rapid reaction significantly delays the loading of O_2 by the red cell. Thus, the uptake of O_2 (or CO) can be regarded as occurring in two stages: (1) diffusion of O_2 through the blood-gas barrier (including the plasma and red cell interior) and (2) reaction of the O_2 with hemoglobin (Figure 3-4). In fact, it is possible to sum the two resultant resistances to produce an overall "diffusion" resistance.

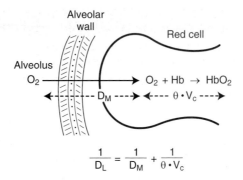

Figure 3-4. The diffusing capacity of the lung (D_L) is made up of two components: that due to the diffusion process itself and that attributable to the time taken for O_2 (or CO) to react with hemoglobin.

We saw that the diffusing capacity of the lung is defined as $D_L = V_{gas}/(P_1 - P_2)$, that is, as the flow of gas divided by a pressure difference. Thus, the inverse of D_L is pressure difference divided by flow and is therefore analogous to electrical resistance. Consequently, the resistance of the blood-gas barrier in Figure 3-4 is shown as $1/D_M$, where M means membrane. Now, the rate of reaction of O_2 (or CO) with hemoglobin can be described by θ, which gives the rate in milliliters per minute of O_2 (or CO) that combine with 1 ml of blood per mm Hg partial pressure of O_2 (or CO). This is analogous to the "diffusing capacity" of 1 ml of blood and, when multiplied by the volume of capillary blood (V_c), gives the effective "diffusing capacity" of the rate of reaction of O_2 with hemoglobin. Again its inverse, $1/(\theta \cdot V_c)$, describes the resistance of this reaction. We can add the resistances offered by the membrane and the blood to obtain the total diffusion resistance. Thus, the complete equation is

$$\frac{1}{D_L} = \frac{1}{D_M} + \frac{1}{\theta \cdot V_c}$$

In practice, the resistances offered by the membrane and blood components are approximately equal, so that a reduction of capillary blood volume by disease can reduce the measured diffusing capacity of the lung. θ for CO is reduced if a subject breathes a high O_2 mixture, because the O_2 competes with the CO for hemoglobin. As a result, the measured diffusing capacity is reduced by O_2 breathing. In fact, it is possible to separately determine D_M and V_c by measuring the diffusing capacity for CO at different alveolar Po_2 values.

Reaction Rates of O_2 and CO with Hemoglobin

- The reaction rate of O_2 is fast, but because so little time is available in the capillary, this rate can become a limiting factor.
- The resistance to the uptake of O_2 attributable to reaction rate is probably about the same as that due to diffusion across the blood-gas barrier.
- The reaction rate of CO can be altered by changing the alveolar P_{O_2}. In this way, the separate contributions of the diffusion properties of the blood-gas barrier and the volume of capillary blood can be derived.

▶ Interpretation of Diffusing Capacity for CO

It is clear that the measured diffusing capacity of the lung for CO depends not only on the area and thickness of the blood-gas barrier but also on the volume of blood in the pulmonary capillaries. Furthermore, in the diseased lung, the measurement is affected by the distribution of diffusion properties, alveolar volume, and capillary blood. For these reasons, the term *transfer factor* is sometimes used (particularly in Europe) to emphasize that the measurement does not solely reflect the diffusion properties of the lung.

▶ CO_2 Transfer Across the Pulmonary Capillary

We have seen that diffusion of CO_2 through tissue is about 20 times faster than that of O_2 because of the much higher solubility of CO_2 (Figure 3-1). At first sight, therefore, it seems unlikely that CO_2 elimination could be affected by diffusion difficulties, and indeed, this has been the general belief. However, the reaction of CO_2 with blood is complex (see Chapter 6), and although there is some uncertainty about the rates of the various reactions, it is possible that a difference between end-capillary blood and alveolar gas can develop if the blood-gas barrier is diseased.

KEY CONCEPTS

1. Fick's law states that the rate of diffusion of a gas through a tissue sheet is proportional to the area of the sheet and the partial pressure difference across it, and inversely proportional to the thickness of the sheet.
2. Examples of diffusion- and perfusion-limited gases are carbon monoxide and nitrous oxide, respectively. Oxygen transfer is normally perfusion limited, but

some diffusion limitation may occur under some conditions, including intense exercise, thickening of the blood-gas barrier, and alveolar hypoxia.
3. The diffusing capacity of the lung is measured using inhaled carbon monoxide. The value increases markedly on exercise.
4. The finite reaction rate of oxygen with hemoglobin can reduce its transfer rate into the blood, and the effect is similar to that of reducing the diffusion rate.
5. Carbon dioxide transfer across the blood-gas barrier is probably not diffusion limited.

QUESTIONS

For each question, choose the one best answer.

1. Using Fick's law of diffusion of gases through a tissue slice, if gas X is 4 times as soluble and 4 times as dense as gas Y, what is the ratio of the diffusion rates of X to Y?

   A. 0.25
   B. 0.5
   C. 2
   D. 4
   E. 8

2. An exercising subject breathes a low concentration of CO in a steady state. If the alveolar P_{CO} is 0.5 mm Hg and the CO uptake is 30 ml·min⁻¹, what is the diffusing capacity of the lung for CO in ml·min⁻¹·mm·Hg⁻¹?

   A. 20
   B. 30
   C. 40
   D. 50
   E. 60

3. In a normal person, doubling the diffusing capacity of the lung would be expected to

   A. Decrease arterial P_{CO_2} during resting breathing.
   B. Increase resting oxygen uptake when the subject breathes 10% oxygen.
   C. Increase the uptake of nitrous oxide during anesthesia.
   D. Increase the arterial P_{O_2} during resting breathing.
   E. Increase maximal oxygen uptake at extreme altitude.

4. If a subject inhales several breaths of a gas mixture containing low concentrations of carbon monoxide and nitrous oxide,

   A. The partial pressures of carbon monoxide in alveolar gas and end-capillary blood will be virtually the same.
   B. The partial pressures of nitrous oxide in alveolar gas and end-capillary blood will be very different.
   C. Carbon monoxide is transferred into the blood along the whole length of the capillary.
   D. Little of the nitrous oxide will be taken up in the early part of the capillary.
   E. The uptake of nitrous oxide can be used to measure the diffusing capacity of the lung.

5. Concerning the diffusing capacity of the lung,

   A. It is best measured with carbon monoxide because this gas diffuses very slowly across the blood-gas barrier.
   B. Diffusion limitation of oxygen transfer during exercise is more likely to occur at sea level than at high altitude.
   C. Breathing oxygen reduces the measured diffusing capacity for carbon monoxide compared with air breathing.
   D. It is decreased by exercise.
   E. It is increased in pulmonary fibrosis, which thickens the blood-gas barrier.

6. The diffusing capacity of the lung for carbon monoxide is increased by

   A. Emphysema, which causes loss of pulmonary capillaries.
   B. Asbestosis, which causes thickening of the blood-gas barrier.
   C. Pulmonary embolism, which cuts off the blood supply to part of the lung.
   D. Exercise in a normal subject.
   E. Severe anemia.

Blood Flow and Metabolism

4

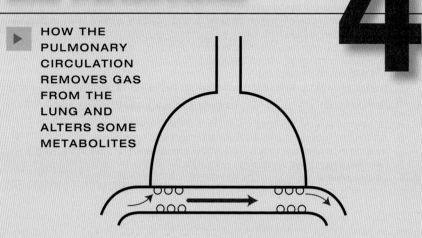

▶ HOW THE
PULMONARY
CIRCULATION
REMOVES GAS
FROM THE
LUNG AND
ALTERS SOME
METABOLITES

We now turn to how the respiratory gases are removed from the lung. First the pressures inside and outside the pulmonary blood vessels are considered, and then pulmonary vascular resistance is introduced. Next, we look at the measurement of total pulmonary blood flow and its uneven distribution caused by gravity. Active control of the circulation is then addressed, followed by fluid balance in the lung. Finally, other functions of the pulmonary circulation are dealt with, particularly the metabolic functions of the lung.

The pulmonary circulation begins at the main pulmonary artery, which receives the mixed venous blood pumped by the right ventricle. This artery then branches successively like the system of airways (Figure 1-3), and, indeed, the pulmonary arteries accompany the airways as far as the terminal bronchioles. Beyond that, they break up to supply the capillary bed that lies in the walls of the alveoli (Figures 1-6 and 1-7). The pulmonary capillaries form a dense network in the alveolar wall that makes an exceedingly efficient arrangement for gas exchange (Figures 1-1, 1-6, and 1-7). So rich is the mesh that some physiologists feel that it is misleading to talk of a network of individual capillary segments, and they prefer to regard the capillary bed as a sheet of flowing blood interrupted in places by posts (Figure 1-6), rather like an underground parking garage. The oxygenated blood is then collected from the capillary bed by the small pulmonary veins that run between the lobules and eventually unite to form the four large veins (in humans), which drain into the left atrium.

At first sight, this circulation appears to be simply a small version of the systemic circulation, which begins at the aorta and ends in the right atrium. However, there are important differences between the two circulations, and confusion frequently results from attempts to emphasize similarities between them.

▶ Pressures Within Pulmonary Blood Vessels

The pressures in the pulmonary circulation are remarkably low. The mean pressure in the main pulmonary artery is only about 15 mm Hg; the systolic and diastolic pressures are about 25 and 8 mm Hg, respectively (Figure 4-1). The pressure is therefore very pulsatile. By contrast, the mean pressure in

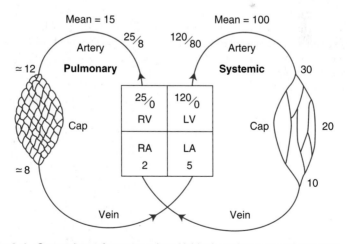

Figure 4-1. Comparison of pressures (mm Hg) in the pulmonary and systemic circulations. Hydrostatic differences modify these.

the aorta is about 100 mm Hg—about six times more than in the pulmonary artery. The pressures in the right and left atriums are not very dissimilar— about 2 and 5 mm Hg, respectively. Thus, the pressure differences from inlet to outlet of the pulmonary and systemic systems are about (15 − 5) = 10 and (100 − 2) = 98 mm Hg, respectively—a factor of 10.

In keeping with these low pressures, the walls of the pulmonary artery and its branches are remarkably thin and contain relatively little smooth muscle (they are easily mistaken for veins). This is in striking contrast to the systemic circulation, where the arteries generally have thick walls and the arterioles in particular have abundant smooth muscle.

The reasons for these differences become clear when the functions of the two circulations are compared. The systemic circulation regulates the supply of blood to various organs, including those which may be far above the level of the heart (the upstretched arm, for example). By contrast, the lung is required to accept the whole of the cardiac output at all times. It is rarely concerned with directing blood from one region to another (an exception is localized alveolar hypoxia; see below), and its arterial pressure is therefore as low as is consistent with lifting blood to the top of the lung. This keeps the work of the right heart as small as is feasible for efficient gas exchange to occur in the lung.

The pressure within the pulmonary capillaries is uncertain. The best evidence suggests that it lies about halfway between pulmonary arterial and venous pressure, and that probably much of the pressure drop occurs within the capillary bed itself. Certainly the distribution of pressures along the pulmonary circulation is far more symmetrical than in its systemic counterpart, where most of the pressure drop is just upstream of the capillaries (Figure 4-1). In addition, the pressure within the pulmonary capillaries varies considerably throughout the lung because of hydrostatic effects (see below).

▶ Pressures Around Pulmonary Blood Vessels

The pulmonary capillaries are unique in that they are virtually surrounded by gas (Figures 1-1 and 1-7). It is true that there is a very thin layer of epithelial cells lining the alveoli, but the capillaries receive little support from this and, consequently, are liable to collapse or distend, depending on the pressures within and around them. The latter is very close to alveolar pressure. (The pressure in the alveoli is usually close to atmospheric pressure; indeed, during breath-holding with the glottis open, the two pressures are identical.) Under some special conditions, the effective pressure around the capillaries is reduced by the surface tension of the fluid lining the alveoli. But usually, the effective pressure is alveolar pressure, and when this rises above the pressure inside the capillaries, they collapse. The pressure difference between the inside and outside of the capillaries is often called the *transmural pressure*.

What is the pressure around the pulmonary arteries and veins? This can be considerably less than alveolar pressure. As the lung expands, these larger

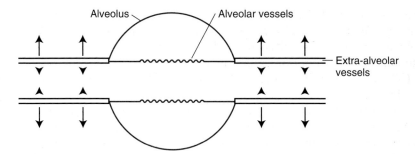

Figure 4-2. "Alveolar" and "extra-alveolar" vessels. The first are mainly the capillaries and are exposed to alveolar pressure. The second are pulled open by the radial traction of the surrounding lung parenchyma, and the effective pressure around them is therefore lower than alveolar pressure.

blood vessels are pulled open by the radial traction of the elastic lung paren-chyma that surrounds them (Figures 4-2 and 4-3). Consequently, the effective pressure around them is low; in fact, there is some evidence that this pressure is even less than the pressure around the whole lung (intrapleural pressure). This paradox can be explained by the mechanical advantage that develops when a relatively rigid structure such as a blood vessel or bronchus is surrounded by a rapidly expanding elastic material such as lung parenchyma. In any event, both the arteries and veins increase their caliber as the lung expands.

The behavior of the capillaries and the larger blood vessels is so different they are often referred to as alveolar and extra-alveolar vessels, respectively (Figure 4-2). Alveolar vessels are exposed to alveolar pressure and include

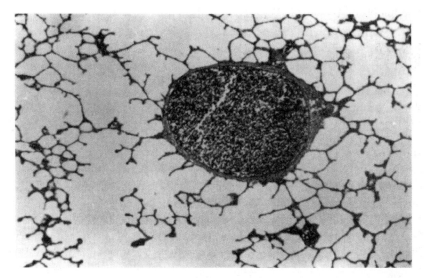

Figure 4-3. Section of lung showing many alveoli and an extra-alveolar vessel (in this case, a small vein) with its perivascular sheath.

the capillaries and the slightly larger vessels in the corners of the alveolar walls. Their caliber is determined by the relationship between alveolar pressure and the pressure within them. Extra-alveolar vessels include all the arteries and veins that run through the lung parenchyma. Their caliber is greatly affected by lung volume because this determines the expanding pull of the parenchyma on their walls. The very large vessels near the hilum are outside the lung substance and are exposed to intrapleural pressure.

Alveolar and Extra-alveolar Vessels

- Alveolar vessels are exposed to alveolar pressure and are compressed if this increases
- Extra-alveolar vessels are exposed to a pressure less than alveolar and are pulled open by the radial traction of the surrounding parenchyma

---

▶ Pulmonary Vascular Resistance

It is useful to describe the resistance of a system of blood vessels as follows:

$$\text{Vascular resistance} = \frac{\text{input pressure} - \text{output pressure}}{\text{blood flow}}$$

This is analogous to electrical resistance, which is (input voltage – output voltage) divided by current. The number for vascular resistance is certainly not a complete description of the pressure-flow properties of the system. For example, the number usually depends on the magnitude of the blood flow. Nevertheless, it often allows a helpful comparison of different circulations or the same circulation under different conditions.

We have seen that the total pressure drop from pulmonary artery to left atrium in the pulmonary circulation is only some 10 mm Hg, against about 100 mm Hg for the systemic circulation. Because the blood flows through the two circulations are virtually identical, it follows that the pulmonary vascular resistance is only one-tenth that of the systemic circulation. The pulmonary blood flow is about 6 liters·min^{-1}, so that, in numbers, the pulmonary vascular resistance is 5 (15 – 5)/6 or about 1.7 mm Hg·liter^{-1}·min.* The high resistance of the systemic circulation is largely caused by very muscular arterioles that allow the regulation of blood flow to various organs of the body. The pulmonary circulation has no such vessels and appears to have as low a resistance as is compatible with distributing the blood in a thin film over a vast area in the alveolar walls.

Although the normal pulmonary vascular resistance is extraordinarily small, it has a remarkable facility for becoming even smaller as the pressure

---

*Cardiologists sometimes express pulmonary vascular resistance in the units dyne·s·cm^{-5}. The normal value is then in the region of 100.

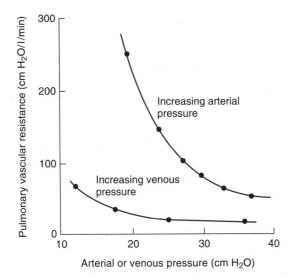

Figure 4-4. Fall in pulmonary vascular resistance as the pulmonary arterial or venous pressure is raised. When the arterial pressure was changed, the venous pressure was held constant at 12 cm water, and when the venous pressure was changed, the arterial pressure was held at 37 cm water. (Data from an excised animal lung preparation.)

within the vessels rises. Figure 4-4 shows that an increase in either pulmonary arterial or venous pressure causes pulmonary vascular resistance to fall. Two mechanisms are responsible for this. Under normal conditions, some capillaries are either closed or open but with no blood flow. As the pressure rises, these vessels begin to conduct blood, thus lowering the overall resistance. This is termed *recruitment* (Figure 4-5) and is apparently the chief mechanism for the fall in pulmonary vascular resistance that occurs as the pulmonary artery pressure is raised from low levels. The reason some vessels are unper-

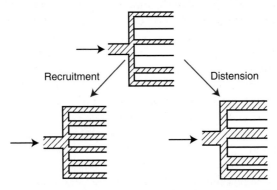

Figure 4-5. Recruitment (opening of previously closed vessels) and distension (increase in caliber of vessels). These are the two mechanisms for the decrease in pulmonary vascular resistance that occurs as vascular pressures are raised.

fused at low perfusing pressures is not fully understood but perhaps is caused by random differences in the geometry of the complex network (Figure 1-6), which result in preferential channels for flow.

At higher vascular pressures, widening of individual capillary segments occurs. This increase in caliber, or *distension*, is hardly surprising in view of the very thin membrane that separates the capillary from the alveolar space (Figure 1-1). Distension is probably chiefly a change in shape of the capillaries from near-flattened to more circular. There is evidence that the capillary wall strongly resists stretching. Distension is apparently the predominant mechanism for the fall in pulmonary vascular resistance at relatively high vascular pressures. However, recruitment and distension often occur together.

Another important determinant of pulmonary vascular resistance is *lung volume*. The caliber of the extra-alveolar vessels (Figure 4-2) is determined by a balance between various forces. As we have seen, they are pulled open as the lung expands. As a result, their vascular resistance is low at large lung volumes. On the other hand, their walls contain smooth muscle and elastic tissue, which resist distension and tend to reduce the caliber of the vessels. Consequently, they have a high resistance when lung volume is low (Figure 4-6). Indeed, if the lung is completely collapsed, the smooth muscle tone of these vessels is so effective that the pulmonary artery pressure has to be raised several centimeters of water above downstream pressure before any flow at all occurs. This is called a *critical opening pressure*.

Is the vascular resistance of the capillaries influenced by lung volume? This depends on whether alveolar pressure changes with respect to the pressure

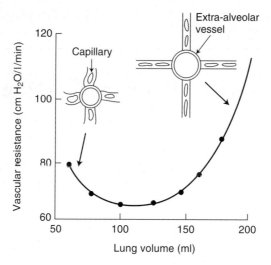

Figure 4-6. Effect of lung volume on pulmonary vascular resistance when the transmural pressure of the capillaries is held constant. At low lung volumes, resistance is high because the extra-alveolar vessels become narrow. At high volumes, the capillaries are stretched, and their caliber is reduced. (Data from an animal lobe preparation.)

inside the capillaries, that is, whether their transmural pressure alters. If alveolar pressure rises with respect to capillary pressure, the vessels tend to be squashed, and their resistance rises. This usually occurs when a normal subject takes a deep inspiration, because the vascular pressures fall. (The heart is surrounded by intrapleural pressure, which falls on inspiration.) However, the pressures in the pulmonary circulation do not remain steady after such a maneuver. An additional factor is that the caliber of the capillaries is reduced at large lung volumes because of stretching and consequent thinning of the alveolar walls. Thus, even if the transmural pressure of the capillaries is not changed with large lung inflations, their vascular resistance increases (Figure 4-6).

Because of the role of smooth muscle in determining the caliber of the extra-alveolar vessels, drugs that cause contraction of the muscle increase pulmonary vascular resistance. These include serotonin, histamine, and norepinephrine. These drugs are particularly effective vasoconstrictors when the lung volume is low and the expanding forces on the vessels are weak. Drugs that can relax smooth muscle in the pulmonary circulation include acetylcholine and isoproterenol.

Pulmonary Vascular Resistance

- Is normally very small
- Decreases on exercise because of recruitment and distension of capillaries
- Increases at high and low lung volumes
- Increases with alveolar hypoxia because of constriction of small pulmonary arteries

▶ Measurement of Pulmonary Blood Flow

The volume of blood passing through the lungs each minute ($\dot{Q}$) can be calculated using the *Fick principle*. This states that the O_2 consumption per minute ($\dot{V}O_2$) measured at the mouth is equal to the amount of O_2 taken up by the blood in the lungs per minute. Because the O_2 concentration in the blood entering the lungs is $C\bar{v}_{O_2}$ and that in the blood leaving is Ca_{O_2}, we have

$$\dot{V}_{O_2} = \dot{Q}(Ca_{O_2} - C\bar{v}_{O_2})$$

or

$$\dot{Q} = \frac{\dot{V}_{O_2}}{Ca_{O_2} - C\bar{v}_{O_2}}$$

$\dot{V}o_2$ is measured by collecting the expired gas in a large spirometer and measuring its O_2 concentration. Mixed venous blood is taken via a catheter in the pulmonary artery, and arterial blood by puncture of the brachial or radial artery. Pulmonary blood flow can also be measured by the indicator dilution technique, in which a dye or other indicator is injected into the venous circulation and its concentration in arterial blood is recorded. Both these methods are of great importance, but they will not be considered in more detail here because they fall within the province of cardiovascular physiology.

▶ Distribution of Blood Flow

So far, we have been assuming that all parts of the pulmonary circulation behave identically. However, considerable inequality of blood flow exists within the upright human lung. This can be shown by a modification of the radioactive xenon method that was used to measure the distribution of ventilation (Figure 2-7). For the measurement of blood flow, the xenon is dissolved in saline and injected into a peripheral vein (Figure 4-7). When it reaches the pulmonary capillaries, it is evolved into alveolar gas because of its low solubility, and the distribution of radioactivity can be measured by counters over the chest during breath-holding.

In the upright human lung, blood flow decreases almost linearly from bottom to top, reaching very low values at the apex (Figure 4-7). This distribution is affected by change of posture and exercise. When the

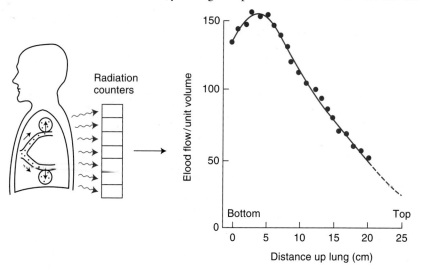

Figure 4-7. Measurement of the distribution of blood flow in the upright human lung, using radioactive xenon. The dissolved xenon is evolved into alveolar gas from the pulmonary capillaries. The units of blood flow are such that if flow were uniform, all values would be 100. Note the small flow at the apex.

subject lies supine, the apical zone blood flow increases, but the basal zone flow remains virtually unchanged, with the result that the distribution from apex to base becomes almost uniform. However, in this posture, blood flow in the posterior (lower or dependent) regions of the lung exceeds flow in the anterior parts. Measurements on subjects suspended upside down show that apical blood flow may exceed basal flow in this position. On mild exercise, both upper and lower zone blood flows increase, and the regional differences become less.

The uneven distribution of blood flow can be explained by the hydrostatic pressure differences within the blood vessels. If we consider the pulmonary arterial system as a continuous column of blood, the difference in pressure between the top and bottom of a lung 30 cm high will be about 30 cm water, or 23 mm Hg. This is a large pressure difference for such a low-pressure system as the pulmonary circulation (Figure 4-1), and its effects on regional blood flow are shown in Figure 4-8.

There may be a region at the top of the lung (*zone 1*) where pulmonary arterial pressure falls below alveolar pressure (normally close to atmospheric pressure). If this occurs, the capillaries are squashed flat, and no flow is possible. Zone 1 does *not* occur under normal conditions, because the pulmonary arterial pressure is just sufficient to raise blood to the top of the lung, but may be present if the arterial pressure is reduced (following severe hemorrhage, for example) or if alveolar pressure is raised (during positive pressure

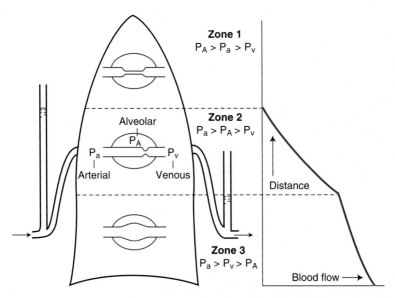

Figure 4-8. Explanation of the uneven distribution of blood flow in the lung, based on the pressures affecting the capillaries. See text for details.

ventilation). This ventilated but unperfused lung is useless for gas exchange and is called *alveolar dead space*.

Farther down the lung (*zone 2*), pulmonary arterial pressure increases because of the hydrostatic effect and now exceeds alveolar pressure. However, venous pressure is still very low and is less than alveolar pressure, which leads to remarkable pressure-flow characteristics. Under these conditions, blood flow is determined by the difference between arterial and alveolar pressures (not the usual arterial-venous pressure difference). Indeed, venous pressure has no influence on flow unless it exceeds alveolar pressure.

This behavior can be modeled with a flexible rubber tube inside a glass chamber (Figure 4-9). When chamber pressure is greater than downstream pressure, the rubber tube collapses at its downstream end, and the pressure inside the tube at this point limits flow. The pulmonary capillary bed is clearly very different from a rubber tube. Nevertheless, the overall behavior is similar and is often called the Starling resistor, sluice, or waterfall effect. Because arterial pressure is increasing down the zone but alveolar pressure is the same throughout the lung, the pressure difference responsible for flow increases. In addition, increasing recruitment of capillaries occurs down this zone.

In *zone 3*, venous pressure now exceeds alveolar pressure, and flow is determined in the usual way by the arterial-venous pressure difference. The increase in blood flow down this region of the lung is apparently caused chiefly by distension of the capillaries. The pressure within them (lying between arterial and venous) increases down the zone while the pressure outside (alveolar) remains constant. Thus, their transmural pressure rises and, indeed, measurements show that their mean width increases. Recruitment of previously closed vessels may also play some part in the increase in blood flow down this zone.

The scheme shown in Figure 4-8 summarizes the role played by the capillaries in determining the distribution of blood flow. At low lung volumes, the

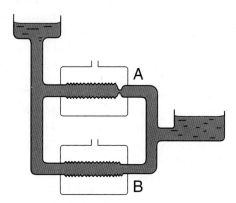

Figure 4-9. Two Starling resistors, each consisting of a thin rubber tube inside a container. When chamber pressure exceeds downstream pressure as in *A*, flow is independent of downstream pressure. However, when downstream pressure exceeds chamber pressure as in *B*, flow is determined by the upstream-downstream difference.

resistance of the extra-alveolar vessels becomes important, and a reduction of regional blood flow is seen, starting first at the base of the lung, where the parenchyma is least expanded (see Figure 7-8). This region of reduced blood flow is sometimes called *zone 4* and can be explained by the narrowing of the extra-alveolar vessels, which occurs when the lung around them is poorly inflated (Figure 4-6).

There are other factors causing unevenness of blood flow in the lung. The complex, partly random arrangement of blood vessels and capillaries (Figure 1-6) causes some inequality of blood flow at any given level in the lung. There is also evidence that blood flow decreases along the acinus, with peripheral parts less well supplied with blood. Some measurements suggest that the peripheral regions of the whole lung receive less blood flow than the central regions. In some animals, some regions of the lung appear to have an intrinsically higher vascular resistance.

▶ Active Control of the Circulation

We have seen that passive factors dominate the vascular resistance and the distribution of flow in the pulmonary circulation under normal conditions. However, a remarkable active response occurs when the Po_2 of alveolar gas is reduced. This is known as *hypoxic pulmonary vasoconstriction* and consists of contraction of smooth muscle in the walls of the small arterioles in the hypoxic region. The precise mechanism of this response is not known, but it occurs in excised isolated lung and so does not depend on central nervous connections. Excised segments of pulmonary artery constrict if their environment is made hypoxic, so there is a local action of the hypoxia on the artery itself. The Po_2 of the alveolar gas, not the pulmonary arterial blood, chiefly determines the response. This can be proved by perfusing a lung with blood of a high Po_2 while keeping the alveolar Po_2 low. Under these conditions, the response occurs.

The vessel wall becomes hypoxic as a result of diffusion of oxygen over the very short distance from the wall to the surrounding alveoli. Recall that a small pulmonary artery is very closely surrounded by alveoli (compare the proximity of alveoli to the small pulmonary vein in Figure 4-3). The stimulus-response curve of this constriction is very nonlinear (Figure 4-10). When the alveolar Po_2 is altered in the region above 100 mm Hg, little change in vascular resistance is seen. However, when the alveolar Po_2 is reduced below approximately 70 mm Hg, marked vasoconstriction may occur, and at a very low Po_2, the local blood flow may be almost abolished.

The mechanism of hypoxic pulmonary vasoconstriction is the subject of a great deal of research. Recent studies show that inhibition of voltage-gated potassium channels and membrane depolarization are involved, leading to increased calcium ion concentrations in the cytoplasm. An increase in cytoplasmic calcium ion concentration is the major trigger for smooth muscle contraction.

Endothelium-derived vasoactive substances play a role. Nitric oxide (NO) has been shown to be an endothelium-derived relaxing factor for blood vessels. It is formed from L-arginine via catalysis by endothelial NO synthase (eNOS) and is a final common pathway for a variety of biological processes. NO activates soluble guanylate cyclase and increases the synthesis of guanosine 3',5'-cyclic monophosphate (cyclic GMP), which leads to smooth muscle relaxation. Inhibitors of NO synthase augment hypoxic pulmonary vasoconstriction in animal preparations, and inhaled NO reduces hypoxic pulmonary vasoconstriction in humans. The required inhaled concentration of NO is extremely low (about 20 ppm), and the gas is very toxic at high concentrations. Disruption of the eNOS gene has been shown to cause pulmonary hypertension in animal models.

Hypoxic Pulmonary Vasoconstriction

- Alveolar hypoxia constricts small pulmonary arteries
- Probably a direct effect of the low P_{O_2} on vascular smooth muscle
- Its release is critical at birth in the transition from placental to air breathing
- Directs blood flow away from poorly ventilated areas of the diseased lung in the adult

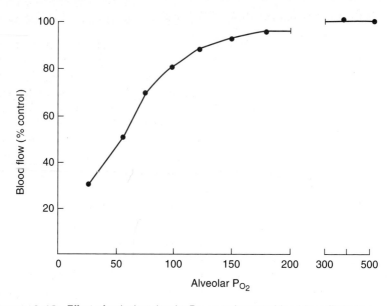

Figure 4-10. Effect of reducing alveolar P_{O_2} on pulmonary blood flow. (Data from anesthetized cat.)

Pulmonary vascular endothelial cells also release potent vasoconstrictors such as endothelin-1 (ET-1) and thromboxane A_2 (TXA_2). Their roles in normal physiology and disease are the subject of intense study. Blockers of endothelin receptors have been used clinically to treat patients with pulmonary hypertension.

Hypoxic vasoconstriction has the effect of directing blood flow away from hypoxic regions of lung. These regions may result from bronchial obstruction, and by diverting blood flow, the deleterious effects on gas exchange are reduced. At high altitude, generalized pulmonary vasoconstriction occurs, leading to a rise in pulmonary arterial pressure. But probably the most important situation in which this mechanism operates is at birth. During fetal life, the pulmonary vascular resistance is very high, partly because of hypoxic vasoconstriction, and only some 15% of the cardiac output goes through the lungs (see Figure 9-5). When the first breath oxygenates the alveoli, the vascular resistance falls dramatically because of relaxation of vascular smooth muscle, and the pulmonary blood flow increases enormously.

Other active responses of the pulmonary circulation have been described. A low blood pH causes vasoconstriction, especially when alveolar hypoxia is present. The autonomic nervous system exerts a weak control, an increase in sympathetic outflow causing stiffening of the walls of the pulmonary arteries and vasoconstriction.

▶ Water Balance in the Lung

Because only 0.3 μm of tissue separates the capillary blood from the air in the lung (Figure 1-1), the problem of keeping the alveoli free of fluid is critical. Fluid exchange across the capillary endothelium obeys Starling's law. The force tending to push fluid *out* of the capillary is the capillary hydrostatic pressure minus the hydrostatic pressure in the interstitial fluid, or $P_c - P_i$. The force tending to pull fluid in is the colloid osmotic pressure of the proteins of the blood minus that of the proteins of the interstitial fluid, or $\pi_c - \pi_i$. This force depends on the reflection coefficient σ, which is a measure of the effectiveness of the capillary wall in preventing the passage of proteins across it. Thus,

$$\text{net fluid out} = K[(P_c - P_i) - \sigma(\pi_c - \pi_i)]$$

where K is a constant called the filtration coefficient.

Unfortunately, the practical use of this equation is limited because of our ignorance of many of the values. The colloid osmotic pressure within the capillary is about 25–28 mm Hg. The capillary hydrostatic pressure is probably about halfway between arterial and venous pressure and is much higher at the bottom of the lung than at the top. The colloid osmotic pressure of the

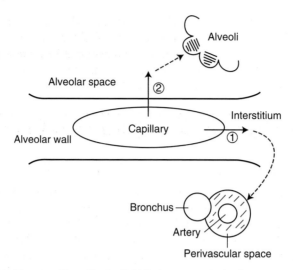

Figure 4-11. Two possible paths for fluid that moves out of pulmonary capillaries. Fluid that enters the interstitium initially finds its way into the perivascular and peribronchial spaces. Later, fluid may cross the alveolar wall, filling alveolar spaces.

interstitial fluid is not known but is about 20 mm Hg in lung lymph. However, this value may be higher than that in the interstitial fluid around the capillaries. The interstitial hydrostatic pressure is unknown, but some measurements show it is substantially below atmospheric pressure. It is probable that the net pressure of the Starling equation is outward, causing a small lymph flow of perhaps 20 ml·h^{-1} in humans under normal conditions.

Where does fluid go when it leaves the capillaries? Figure 4-11 shows that fluid that leaks out into the interstitium of the alveolar wall tracks through the interstitial space to the perivascular and peribronchial space within the lung. Numerous lymphatics run in the perivascular spaces, and these help to transport the fluid to the hilar lymph nodes. In addition, the pressure in these perivascular spaces is low, thus forming a natural sump for the drainage of fluid (compare Figure 4-2). The earliest form of pulmonary edema[†] is characterized by engorgement of these peribronchial and perivascular spaces and is known as interstitial edema. The rate of lymph flow from the lung increases considerably if the capillary pressure is raised over a long period.

In a later stage of pulmonary edema, fluid may cross the alveolar epithelium into the alveolar spaces (Figure 4-11). When this occurs, the alveoli fill with fluid one by one, and because they are then unventilated, no oxygenation of the blood passing through them is possible. What prompts fluid to start moving across into the alveolar spaces is not known, but it may be that

---

[†]For a more extensive discussion of pulmonary edema, see the companion volume, JB West, *Pulmonary Pathophysiology: The Essentials*, 7th ed. (Baltimore, MD: Lippincott Williams & Wilkins, 2007).

this occurs when the maximal drainage rate through the interstitial space is exceeded and the pressure there rises too high. Fluid that reaches the alveolar spaces is actively pumped out by a sodium-potassium ATPase pump in epithelial cells. Alveolar edema is much more serious than interstitial edema because of the interference with pulmonary gas exchange.

▶ Other Functions of the Pulmonary Circulation

The chief function of the pulmonary circulation is to move blood to and from the blood-gas barrier so that gas exchange can occur. However, it has other important functions. One is to act as a reservoir for blood. We saw that the lung has a remarkable ability to reduce its pulmonary vascular resistance as its vascular pressures are raised through the mechanisms of recruitment and distension (Figure 4-5). The same mechanisms allow the lung to increase its blood volume with relatively small rises in pulmonary arterial or venous pressures. This occurs, for example, when a subject lies down after standing. Blood then drains from the legs into the lung.

Another function of the lung is to filter blood. Small blood thrombi are removed from the circulation before they can reach the brain or other vital organs. Many white blood cells are trapped by the lung and later released, although the value of this is not clear.

▶ Metabolic Functions of the Lung

The lung has important metabolic functions in addition to gas exchange. A number of vasoactive substances are metabolized by the lung (Table 4-1). Because the lung is the only organ except the heart that receives the whole circulation, it is uniquely suited to modifying bloodborne substances. A substantial fraction of all the vascular endothelial cells in the body are located in the lung. The metabolic functions of the vascular endothelium are only briefly dealt with here because many fall within the province of pharmacology.

The only known example of biological activation by passage through the pulmonary circulation is the conversion of the relatively inactive polypeptide angiotensin I to the potent vasoconstrictor angiotensin II. The latter, which is up to 50 times more active than its precursor, is unaffected by passage through the lung. The conversion of angiotensin I is catalyzed by angiotensin-converting enzyme, or ACE, which is located in small pits in the surface of the capillary endothelial cells.

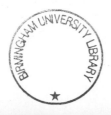

Table 4.1	Fate of Substances in the Pulmonary Circulation
Substance	**Fate**
Peptides	
Angiotensin I	Converted to angiotensin II by ACE
Angiotensin II	Unaffected
Vasporessin	Unaffected
Bradykinin	Up to 80% inactivated
Amines	
Serotonin	Almost completely removed
Norepinephrine	Up to 30% removed
Histamine	Not affected
Dopamine	Not affected
Arachidonic acid metabolites	
Prostaglandins E_2 and $F_{2\alpha}$	Almost completely removed
Prostaglandin A_2	Not affected
Prostacyclin (PGI_2)	Not affected
Leukotrienes	Almost completely removed

Many vasoactive substances are completely or partially inactivated during passage through the lung. Bradykinin is largely inactivated (up to 80%), and the enzyme responsible is ACE. The lung is the major site of inactivation of serotonin (5-hydroxytryptamine), but this is not by enzymatic degradation but by an uptake and storage process (Table 4-1). Some of the serotonin may be transferred to platelets in the lung or stored in some other way and released during anaphylaxis. The prostaglandins E_1, E_2, and $F_{2\alpha}$ are also inactivated in the lung, which is a rich source of the responsible enzymes. Norepinephrine is also taken up by the lung to some extent (up to 30%). Histamine appears not to be affected by the intact lung but is readily inactivated by slices.

Some vasoactive materials pass through the lung without significant gain or loss of activity. These include epinephrine, prostaglandins A_1 and A_2, angiotensin II, and vasopressin (ADH).

Several vasoactive and bronchoactive substances are metabolized in the lung and may be released into the circulation under certain conditions. Important among these are the arachidonic acid metabolites (Figure 4-12). Arachidonic acid is formed through the action of the enzyme phospholipase A_2 on phospholipid bound to cell membranes. There are two major synthetic pathways, the initial reactions being catalyzed by the enzymes lipoxygenase and cyclooxygenase, respectively. The first produces the leukotrienes, which include the mediator originally described as slow-reacting substance of anaphylaxis (SRS-A). These compounds cause airway constriction and may have an important role in asthma.[‡] Other leukotrienes are involved in inflammatory responses.

The prostaglandins are potent vasoconstrictors or vasodilators. Prostaglandin E_2 plays an important role in the fetus because it helps to relax the

[‡]For more details, see JB West, *Pulmonary Pathophysiology: The Essentials*, 7th ed. (Baltimore, MD: Lippincott Williams & Wilkins, 2007).

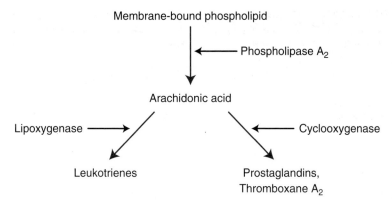

Figure 4-12. Two pathways of arachidonic acid metabolism. The leukotrienes are generated by the lipoxygenase pathway, whereas the prostaglandins and thromboxane A_2 come from the cyclooxygenase pathway.

patent ductus arteriosus. Prostaglandins also affect platelet aggregation and are active in other systems, such as the kallikrein-kinin clotting cascade. They also may have a role in the bronchoconstriction of asthma.

There is also evidence that the lung plays a role in the clotting mechanism of blood under normal and abnormal conditions. For example, there are a large number of mast cells containing heparin in the interstitium. In addition, the lung is able to secrete special immunoglobulins, particularly IgA, in the bronchial mucus that contribute to its defenses against infection.

Synthetic functions of the lung include the synthesis of phospholipids such as dipalmitoyl phosphatidylcholine, which is a component of pulmonary surfactant (see Chapter 7). Protein synthesis is also clearly important because collagen and elastin form the structural framework of the lung. Under some conditions, proteases are apparently liberated from leukocytes in the lung, causing breakdown of collagen and elastin, and this may result in emphysema. Another significant area is carbohydrate metabolism, especially the elaboration of mucopolysaccharides of bronchial mucus.

KEY CONCEPTS

1. The pressures within the pulmonary circulation are much lower than in the systemic circulation. Also the capillaries are exposed to alveolar pressure, whereas the pressures around the extra-alveolar vessels are lower.
2. Pulmonary vascular resistance is low and falls even more when cardiac output increases because of recruitment and distension of the capillaries. Pulmonary vascular resistance increases at very low or high lung volumes.

3. Blood flow is unevenly distributed in the upright lung. There is a higher flow at the base than at the apex as a result of gravity. If capillary pressure is less than alveolar pressure at the top of the lung, the capillaries collapse and there is no blood flow (zone 1). There is also uneven blood flow at any given level in the lung because of random variations of the blood vessels.
4. Hypoxic pulmonary vasoconstriction reduces the blood flow to poorly ventilated regions of the lung. Release of this mechanism is responsible for a large increase in blood flow to the lung at birth.
5. Fluid movement across the capillary endothelium is governed by the Starling equilibrium.
6. The pulmonary circulation has many metabolic functions, notably the conversion of angiotensin I to angiotensin II by angiotensin-converting enzyme.

QUESTIONS

For each question, choose the one best answer.

1. The ratio of total systemic vascular resistance to pulmonary vascular resistance is about

   A. 2: 1
   B. 3: 1
   C. 5: 1
   D. 10: 1
   E. 20: 1

2. Concerning the extra-alveolar vessels of the lung,

   A. Tension in the surrounding alveolar walls tends to narrow them.
   B. Their walls contain smooth muscle and elastic tissue.
   C. They are exposed to alveolar pressure.
   D. Their constriction in response to alveolar hypoxia mainly takes place in the veins.
   E. Their caliber is reduced by lung inflation.

3. A patient with pulmonary vascular disease has mean pulmonary arterial and venous pressures of 55 and 5 mm Hg, respectively, while the cardiac output is 3 liters·min^{-1}. What is his pulmonary vascular resistance in mm Hg·liters^{-1}·min?

   A. 0.5
   B. 1.7
   C. 2.5
   D. 5
   F. 17

4. The fall in pulmonary vascular resistance on exercise is caused by

   A. Decrease in pulmonary arterial pressure.
   B. Decrease in pulmonary venous pressure.
   C. Increase in alveolar pressure.
   D. Distension of pulmonary capillaries.
   E. Alveolar hypoxia.

5. In a measurement of cardiac output using the Fick principle, the O_2 concentrations of mixed venous and arterial blood are 16 and 20 ml· 100 ml^{-1}, respectively, and the O_2 consumption is 300 ml·min^{-1}. The cardiac output in liters·min^{-1} is

A. 2.5
B. 5
C. 7.5
D. 10
E. 75

6. In zone 2 of the lung,

A. Alveolar pressure exceeds arterial pressure.
B. Venous pressure exceeds alveolar pressure.
C. Venous pressure exceeds arterial pressure.
D. Blood flow is determined by arterial pressure minus alveolar pressure.
E. Blood flow is unaffected by arterial pressure.

7. Pulmonary vascular resistance is reduced by

A. Removal of one lung.
B. Breathing a 10% oxygen mixture.
C. Exhaling from functional residual capacity to residual volume.
D. Acutely increasing pulmonary venous pressure.
E. Mechanically ventilating the lung with positive pressure.

8. Hypoxic pulmonary vasoconstriction

A. Depends more on the P_{O_2} of mixed venous blood than alveolar gas.
B. Is released in the transition from placental to air respiration.
C. Involves CO_2 uptake in vascular smooth muscle.
D. Partly diverts blood flow from well-ventilated regions of diseased lungs.
E. Is increased by inhaling low concentrations of nitric oxide.

9. If the pressures in the capillaries and interstitial space at the top of the lung are 3 and 0 mm Hg, respectively, and the colloid osmotic pressures of the blood and interstitial fluid are 25 and 5 mm Hg, respectively, what is the net pressure in mm Hg moving fluid into the capillaries?

A. 17
B. 20
C. 23
D. 27
E. 33

10. The metabolic functions of the lung include

A. Converting angiotensin II to angiotensin I.
B. Producing bradykinin.
C. Secreting serotonin.
D. Removing leukotrienes.
E. Generating erythropoietin.

Ventilation-Perfusion Relationships

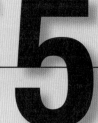

5

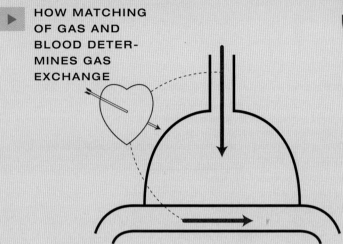

This chapter is devoted to the primary function of the lung, that is, gas exchange. First, a theoretical ideal lung is considered. Then we review three mechanisms of hypoxemia: hypoventilation, diffusion limitation, and shunt. The difficult concept of ventilation-perfusion inequality is then introduced, and to illustrate this the regional differences of gas exchange in the upright human lung are described. Then we examine how ventilation-perfusion inequality impairs overall gas exchange. It is emphasized that this is true not only of oxygen but also of carbon dioxide. Methods of measuring ventilation-perfusion inequality are then briefly discussed.

So far we have considered the movement of air to and from the blood-gas interface, the diffusion of gas across it, and the movement of blood to and from the barrier. It would be natural to assume that if all these processes were adequate, normal gas exchange within the lung would be assured. Unfortunately, this is not so because the matching of ventilation and blood flow within various regions of the lung is critical for adequate gas exchange. Indeed, mismatching of ventilation and blood flow is responsible for most of the defective gas exchange in pulmonary diseases.

In this chapter, we shall look closely at the important (but difficult) subject of how the relations between ventilation and blood flow determine gas exchange. First, however, we shall examine two relatively simple causes of impairment of gas exchange—hypoventilation and shunt. Because all of these situations result in *hypoxemia*, that is, in an abnormally low Po_2 in arterial blood, it is useful to take a preliminary look at normal O_2 transfer.

▶ Oxygen Transport from Air to Tissues

Figure 5-1 shows how the Po_2 falls as the gas moves from the atmosphere in which we live to the mitochondria where it is utilized. The Po_2 of air is 20.93% of the total dry gas pressure (that is, excluding water vapor). At sea level, the barometric pressure is 760 mm Hg, and at the body temperature of 37°C, the water vapor pressure of moist inspired gas (which is fully saturated with water vapor) is 47 mm Hg. Thus, the Po_2 of inspired air is (20.93/100) × (760 – 47), or 149 mm Hg (say 150).

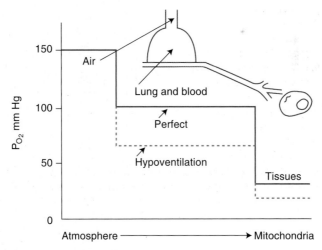

Figure 5-1. Scheme of the O_2 partial pressures from air to tissues. The *solid line* shows a hypothetical perfect situation, and the *broken line* depicts hypoventilation. Hypoventilation depresses the Po_2 in the alveolar gas and, therefore, in the tissues.

Figure 5-1 is drawn for a hypothetical perfect lung, and it shows that by the time the O_2 has reached the alveoli, the Po_2 has fallen to about 100 mm Hg, that is, by one-third. This is because the Po_2 of alveolar gas is determined by a balance between two processes: the removal of O_2 by pulmonary capillary blood on the one hand and its continual replenishment by alveolar ventilation on the other. (Strictly, alveolar ventilation is not continuous but is breath by breath. However, the fluctuation in alveolar Po_2 with each breath is only about 3 mm Hg, because the tidal volume is small compared with the volume of gas in the lung, so the process can be regarded as continuous.) The rate of removal of O_2 from the lung is governed by the O_2 consumption of the tissues and varies little under resting conditions. In practice, therefore, the alveolar Po_2 is largely determined by the level of alveolar ventilation. The same applies to the alveolar Pco_2, which is normally about 40 mm Hg.

Four Causes of Hypoxemia

- Hypoventilation
- Diffusion limitation
- Shunt
- Ventilation-perfusion inequality

When the systemic arterial blood reaches the tissue capillaries, O_2 diffuses to the mitochondria, where the Po_2 is much lower. The "tissue" Po_2 probably differs considerably throughout the body, and in some cells at least, the Po_2 is as low as 1 mm Hg. However, the lung is an essential link in the chain of O_2 transport, and any decrease of Po_2 in arterial blood must result in a lower tissue Po_2, other things being equal. For the same reasons, impaired pulmonary gas exchange causes a rise in tissue Pco_2.

▶ Hypoventilation

We have seen that the level of alveolar Po_2 is determined by a balance between the rate of removal of O_2 by the blood (which is set by the metabolic demands of the tissues) and the rate of replenishment of O_2 by alveolar ventilation. Thus, if the alveolar ventilation is abnormally low, the alveolar Po_2 falls. For similar reasons, the Pco_2 rises. This is known as hypoventilation (Figure 5-1).

Causes of hypoventilation include such drugs as morphine and barbiturates that depress the central drive to the respiratory muscles, damage to the chest wall or paralysis of the respiratory muscles, and a high resistance to breathing (for example, very dense gas at great depth underwater). Hypoventilation always causes an increased alveolar and, therefore, arterial P_{CO_2}. The relationship between alveolar ventilation and P_{CO_2} was derived on p. 20 in the alveolar ventilation equation:

$$P_{CO_2} = \frac{\dot{V}_{CO_2}}{\dot{V}_A} \times K$$

where $\dot{V}_{CO_2}$ is the CO_2 production, $\dot{V}_A$ is the alveolar ventilation, and K is a constant. This means that if the alveolar ventilation is halved, the P_{CO_2} is doubled, once a steady state has been established.

Hypoventilation

- Always increases the alveolar and arterial P_{CO_2}
- Decreases the P_{O_2} unless additional O_2 is inspired
- Hypoxemia is easy to reverse by adding O_2 to the inspired gas

The relationship between the fall in P_{O_2} and the rise in P_{CO_2} that occurs in hypoventilation can be calculated from the *alveolar gas equation* if we know the composition of inspired gas and the respiratory exchange ratio R. The latter is given by the CO_2 production/O_2 consumption and is determined by the metabolism of the tissues in a steady state. It is sometimes known as the respiratory quotient. A simplified form of the alveolar gas equation is

$$P_{A_{O_2}} = P_{I_{O_2}} - \frac{P_{A_{CO_2}}}{R} + F$$

where F is a small correction factor (typically about 2 mm Hg for air breathing), which we can ignore. This equation shows that if R has its normal value of 0.8, the fall in alveolar P_{O_2} is slightly greater than is the rise in P_{CO_2} during hypoventilation. The full version of the equation is given in Appendix A.

Hypoventilation always reduces the alveolar and arterial P_{O_2} except when the subject breathes an enriched O_2 mixture. In this case, the added amount of O_2 per breath can easily make up for the reduced flow of inspired gas (try question 3 on p. 75).

If alveolar ventilation is suddenly increased (for example, by voluntary hyperventilation), it may take several minutes for the alveolar P_{O_2} and P_{CO_2} to assume their new steady-state values. This is because of the different O_2 and CO_2 stores in the body. The CO_2 stores are much greater than the O_2 stores because of the large amount of CO_2 in the form of bicarbonate in the blood and interstitial fluid (see Chapter 6). Therefore, the alveolar P_{CO_2} takes longer to come to equilibrium, and during the nonsteady state, the R value of expired gas is high as the CO_2 stores are washed out. Opposite changes occur with the onset of hypoventilation.

► Diffusion

Figure 5-1 shows that in a perfect lung, the Po$_2$ of arterial blood would be the same as that in alveolar gas. In real life, this is not so. One reason is that although the Po$_2$ of the blood rises closer and closer to that of alveolar gas as the blood traverses the pulmonary capillary (Figure 3-3), it can never quite reach it. Under normal conditions, the Po$_2$ difference between alveolar gas and end-capillary blood resulting from incomplete diffusion is immeasurably small but is shown schematically in Figure 5-2. As we have seen, the difference can become larger during exercise, or when the blood-gas barrier is thickened, or if a low O$_2$ mixture is inhaled (Figure 3-3B).

► Shunt

Another reason why the Po$_2$ of arterial blood is less than that in alveolar gas is shunted blood. *Shunt* refers to blood that enters the arterial system without going through ventilated areas of the lung. In the normal lung, some of the bronchial artery blood is collected by the pulmonary veins after it has perfused the bronchi and its O$_2$ has been partly depleted. Another source is a small amount of coronary venous blood that drains directly into the cavity of the left ventricle through the thebesian veins. The effect of the addition of this poorly oxygenated blood is to depress the arterial Po$_2$. Some patients have an abnormal vascular connection between a small pulmonary artery and vein (pulmonary arteriovenous fistula). In patients with heart disease, there

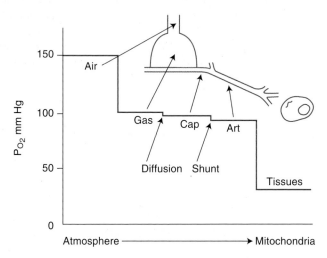

Figure 5-2. Scheme of O$_2$ transfer from air to tissues showing the depression of arterial Po$_2$ caused by diffusion and shunt.

may be a direct addition of venous blood to arterial blood across a defect between the right and left sides of the heart.

When the shunt is caused by the addition of mixed venous blood to blood draining from the capillaries, it is possible to calculate the amount of the shunt flow (Figure 5-3). The total amount of O_2 leaving the system is the total blood flow $\dot{Q}_T$ multiplied by the O_2 concentration in the arterial blood Ca_{O_2}, or $\dot{Q}_T \times Ca_{O_2}$. This must equal the sum of the amounts of O_2 in the shunted blood, $\dot{Q}_S \times C\bar{v}_{O_2}$, and end-capillary blood, $(\dot{Q}_T - \dot{Q}_S) \times Cc'_O$. Thus,

$$\dot{Q}_T \times Ca_{O_2} = \dot{Q}_S \times C\bar{v}_{O_2} + (\dot{Q}_T - \dot{Q}_S) \times Cc'_{O_2}$$

Rearranging gives

$$\frac{\dot{Q}_S}{\dot{Q}_T} = \frac{Cc'_{O_2} - Ca_{O_2}}{Cc'_{O_2} - C\bar{v}_{O_2}}$$

The O_2 concentration of end-capillary blood is usually calculated from the alveolar P_{O_2} and the oxygen dissociation curve (see Chapter 6).

When the shunt is caused by blood that does not have the same O_2 concentration as mixed venous blood (for example, bronchial vein blood), it is generally not possible to calculate its true magnitude. However, it is often useful to calculate an "as if" shunt, that is, what the shunt *would* be if the observed depression of arterial O_2 concentration were caused by the addition of mixed venous blood.

An important feature of a shunt is that the hypoxemia cannot be abolished by giving the subject 100% O_2 to breathe. This is because the shunted blood that bypasses ventilated alveoli is never exposed to the higher alveolar P_{O_2}, so it continues to depress the arterial P_{O_2}. However, some elevation of the arterial P_{O_2} occurs because of the O_2 added to the capillary blood of ventilated lung. Most of the added O_2 is in the dissolved form, rather than attached to hemoglobin, because the blood that is perfusing ventilated alveoli is nearly

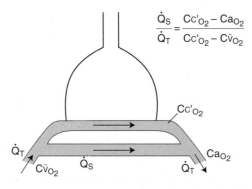

Figure 5-3. Measurement of shunt flow. The oxygen carried in the arterial blood equals the sum of the oxygen carried in the capillary blood and that in the shunted blood (see text).

fully saturated (see Chapter 6). Giving the subject 100% O_2 to breathe is a very sensitive measurement of shunt because when the Po_2 is high, a small depression of arterial O_2 concentration causes a relatively large fall in Po_2 due to the almost flat slope of the O_2 dissociation curve in this region (Figure 5-4).

A shunt usually does not result in a raised Pco_2 in arterial blood, even though the shunted blood is rich in CO_2. The reason is that the chemoreceptors sense any elevation of arterial Pco_2 and they respond by increasing the ventilation. This reduces the Pco_2 of the unshunted blood until the arterial Pco_2 is normal. Indeed, in some patients with a shunt, the arterial Pco_2 is low because the hypoxemia increases respiratory drive (see Chapter 8).

Shunt

- Hypoxemia responds poorly to added inspired O_2
- When 100% O_2 is inspired, the arterial Po_2 does not rise to the expected level—a useful diagnostic test
- If the shunt is caused by mixed venous blood, its size can be calculated from the shunt equation

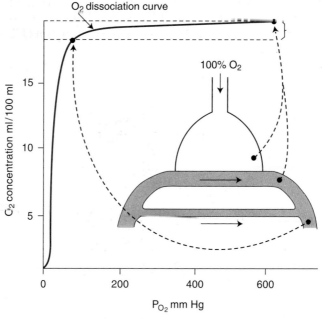

Figure 5-4. Depression of arterial Po_2 by shunt during 100% O_2 breathing. The addition of a small amount of shunted blood with its low O_2 concentration greatly reduces the Po_2 of arterial blood. This is because the O_2 dissociation curve is nearly flat when the Po_2 is very high.

▶ The Ventilation-Perfusion Ratio

So far, we have considered three of the four causes of hypoxemia: hypoventilation, diffusion, and shunt. We now come to the last cause, which is both the most common and the most difficult to understand, namely, ventilation-perfusion inequality. It turns out that if ventilation and blood flow are mismatched in various regions of the lung, impairment of both O_2 and CO_2 transfer results. The key to understanding how this happens is the ventilation-perfusion ratio.

Consider a model of a lung unit (Figure 2-1) in which the uptake of O_2 is being mimicked using dye and water (Figure 5-5). Powdered dye is continuously poured into the unit to represent the addition of O_2 by alveolar ventilation. Water is pumped continuously through the unit to represent the blood flow that removes the O_2. A stirrer mixes the alveolar contents, a process normally accomplished by gaseous diffusion. The key question is: What determines the concentration of dye (or O_2) in the alveolar compartment and, therefore, in the effluent water (or blood)?

It is clear that both the rate at which the dye is added (ventilation) and the rate at which water is pumped (blood flow) will affect the concentration of dye in the model. What may not be intuitively clear is that the concentration of dye is determined by the ratio of these rates. In other words, if dye is added at the rate of V g·min^{-1} and water is pumped through at Q liters·min^{-1},

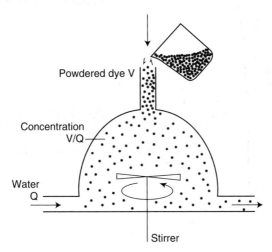

Figure 5-5. Model to illustrate how the ventilation-perfusion ratio determines the P_{O_2} in a lung unit. Powdered dye is added by ventilation at the rate V and removed by blood flow Q to represent the factors controlling alveolar P_{O_2}. The concentration of dye is given by V/Q.

the concentration of dye in the alveolar compartment and effluent water is V/Q g·liter^{-1}.

In exactly the same way, the concentration of O_2 (or, better, Po_2) in any lung unit is determined by the ratio of ventilation to blood flow. This is true not only for O_2 but CO_2, N_2, and any other gas that is present under steady-state conditions. This is why the ventilation-perfusion ratio plays such a key role in pulmonary gas exchange.

▶ Effect of Altering the Ventilation-Perfusion Ratio of a Lung Unit

Let us take a closer look at the way alterations in the ventilation-perfusion ratio of a lung unit affect its gas exchange. Figure 5-6A shows the Po_2 and Pco_2 in a unit with a normal ventilation-perfusion ratio (about 1, see Figure 2-1). The inspired air has a Po_2 of 150 mm Hg (Figure 5-1) and a Pco_2 of 0. The mixed venous blood entering the unit has a Po_2 of 40 mm Hg and a Pco_2 of 45 mm Hg. The alveolar Po_2 of 100 mm Hg is determined by a balance between the addition of O_2 by ventilation and its removal by blood flow. The normal alveolar Pco_2 of 40 mm Hg is set similarly.

Now suppose that the ventilation-perfusion ratio of the unit is gradually reduced by obstructing its ventilation, leaving its blood flow unchanged (Figure 5-6B). It is clear that the O_2 in the unit will fall and the CO_2

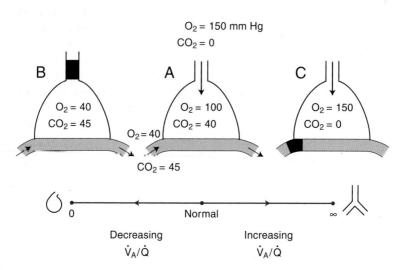

Figure 5-6. Effect of altering the ventilation-perfusion ratio on the Po_2 and Pco_2 in a lung unit.

will rise, although the relative changes of these two are not immediately obvious.* However, we can easily predict what will eventually happen when the ventilation is completely abolished (ventilation-perfusion ratio of 0). Now the O_2 and CO_2 of alveolar gas and end-capillary blood must be the same as those of mixed venous blood. (In practice, completely obstructed units eventually collapse, but we can neglect such long-term effects at the moment.) Note that we are assuming that what happens in one lung unit out of a very large number does not affect the composition of the mixed venous blood.

Suppose instead that the ventilation-perfusion ratio is increased by gradually obstructing blood flow (Figure 5-6C). Now the O_2 rises and the CO_2 falls, eventually reaching the composition of inspired gas when blood flow is abolished (ventilation-perfusion ratio of infinity). Thus, as the ventilation-perfusion ratio of the unit is altered, its gas composition approaches that of mixed venous blood or inspired gas.

A convenient way of depicting these changes is to use the O_2-CO_2 diagram (Figure 5-7). In this, Po_2 is plotted on the X axis, and Pco_2 is plotted on the Y axis. First, locate the normal alveolar gas composition, point A (Po_2 = 100, Pco_2 = 40). If we assume that blood equilibrates with alveolar gas at the end of the capillary (Figure 3-3), this point can equally well represent the end-capillary blood. Next find the mixed venous point $\bar{v}$ (Po_2 = 40, Pco_2 = 45). The bar above v means "mixed" or "mean." Finally, find the inspired point I (Po_2 = 150, Pco_2 = 0). Also, note the similarities between Figures 5-6 and 5-7.

The line joining $\bar{v}$ to I passing through A shows the changes in alveolar gas (and end-capillary blood) composition that can occur when the ventilation-perfusion ratio is either decreased below normal (A → $\bar{v}$) or increased above normal (A → I). Indeed, this line indicates *all* the possible alveolar gas compositions in a lung that is supplied with gas of composition I and blood of composition $\bar{v}$. For example, such a lung could not contain an alveolus with a Po_2 of 70 and Pco_2 of 30 mm Hg, because this point does not lie on the ventilation-perfusion line. However, this alveolar composition *could* exist if the mixed venous blood or inspired gas were changed so that the line then passed through this point.

---

*The alveolar gas equation is not applicable here because the respiratory exchange ratio is not constant. The appropriate equation is

$$\frac{\dot{V}_A}{\dot{Q}} = 8.63 \; R \; \frac{Ca_{O_2} - C\bar{v}_{O_2}}{Pa_{CO_2}}$$

This is called the ventilation-perfusion ratio equation.

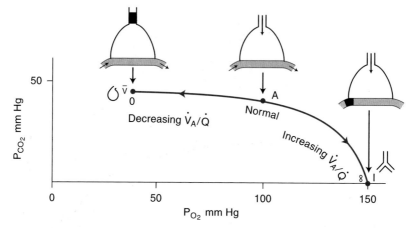

Figure 5-7. O_2-CO_2 diagram showing a ventilation-perfusion ratio line. The P_{O_2} and P_{CO_2} of a lung unit move along this line from the mixed venous point to the inspired gas point I as the ventilation-perfusion ratio is increased (compare Figure 5-6).

▶ Regional Gas Exchange in the Lung

The way in which the ventilation-perfusion ratio of a lung unit determines its gas exchange can be graphically illustrated by looking at the differences that occur down the upright lung. We saw in Figures 2-7 and 4-7 that ventilation increases slowly from top to bottom of the lung and blood flow increases more rapidly (Figure 5-8). As a consequence, the ventilation-perfusion ratio

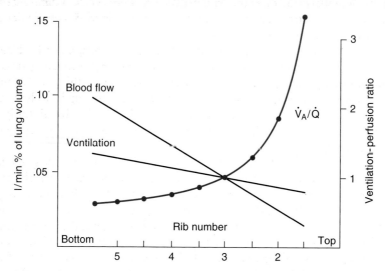

Figure 5-8. Distribution of ventilation and blood flow down the upright lung (compare Figures 2-7 and 4-7). Note that the ventilation-perfusion ratio decreases down the lung.

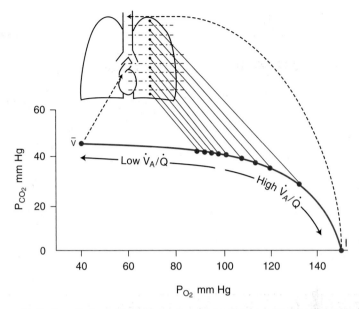

Figure 5-9. Result of combining the pattern of ventilation-perfusion ratio inequality shown in Figure 5-8 with the effects of this on gas exchange as shown in Figure 5-7. Note that the high ventilation-perfusion ratio at the apex results in a high Po_2 and low Pco_2 there. The opposite is seen at the base.

is abnormally high at the top of the lung (where the blood flow is minimal) and much lower at the bottom. We can now use these regional differences in ventilation-perfusion ratio on an O_2-CO_2 diagram (Figure 5-7) to depict the resulting differences in gas exchange.

Figure 5-9 shows the upright lung divided into imaginary horizontal "slices," each of which is located on the ventilation-perfusion line by its own ventilation-perfusion ratio. This ratio is high at the apex, so this point is found toward the right end of the line, whereas the base of the lung is to the left of normal (compare Figure 5-7). It is clear that the Po_2 of the alveoli (horizontal axis) decreases markedly down the lung, whereas the Pco_2 (vertical axis) increases much less.

Figure 5-10 illustrates the values that can be read off a diagram like Figure 5-9. (Of course, there will be variations between individuals; the chief aim of this approach is to describe the principles underlying gas exchange.) Note first that the volume of the lung in the slices is less near the apex than the base. Ventilation is less at the top than the bottom, but the differences in blood flow are more marked. Consequently, the ventilation-perfusion ratio decreases down the lung, and all the differences in gas exchange follow from this. Note that the Po_2 changes by over 40 mm Hg, whereas the difference in Pco_2 between apex and base is much less. (Incidentally, the high Po_2 at

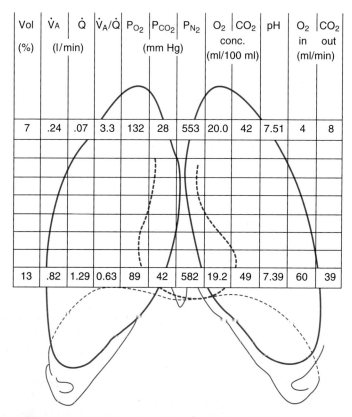

Vol (%)	V̇A (l/min)	Q̇	V̇A/Q̇	PO₂	PCO₂	PN₂ (mm Hg)	O₂ conc.	CO₂ (ml/100 ml)	pH	O₂ in	CO₂ out (ml/min)
7	.24	.07	3.3	132	28	553	20.0	42	7.51	4	8
13	.82	1.29	0.63	89	42	582	19.2	49	7.39	60	39

Figure 5-10. Regional differences in gas exchange down the normal lung. Only the apical and basal values are shown for clarity.

the apex probably accounts for the preference of adult tuberculosis for this region because it provides a more favorable environment for this organism.) The variation in P_{N_2} is, in effect, by default because the total pressure in the alveolar gas is the same throughout the lung.

The regional differences in P_{O_2} and P_{CO_2} imply differences in the end-capillary concentrations of these gases, which can be obtained from the appropriate dissociation curves (Chapter 6). Note the surprisingly large difference in pH down the lung, which reflects the considerable variation in P_{CO_2} of the blood. The minimal contribution to overall O_2 uptake made by the apex can be mainly attributed to the very low blood flow there. The difference in CO_2 output between apex and base is much less because this can be shown to be more closely related to ventilation. As a result, the respiratory exchange ratio (CO_2 output/O_2 uptake) is higher at the apex than at the base. On exercise, when the distribution of blood flow becomes more uniform, the apex assumes a larger share of the O_2 uptake.

▶ Effect of Ventilation-Perfusion Inequality on Overall Gas Exchange

Although the regional differences in gas exchange discussed above are of interest, more important to the body as a whole is whether uneven ventilation and blood flow affect the overall gas exchange of the lung, that is, its ability to take up O_2 and put out CO_2. It turns out that a lung with ventilation-perfusion inequality is not able to transfer as much O_2 and CO_2 as a lung that is uniformly ventilated and perfused, other things being equal. Or if the same amounts of gas are being transferred (because these are set by the metabolic demands of the body), the lung with ventilation-perfusion inequality cannot maintain as high an arterial Po_2 or as low an arterial Pco_2 as a homogeneous lung, again other things being equal.

The reason why a lung with uneven ventilation and blood flow has difficulty oxygenating arterial blood can be illustrated by looking at the differences down the upright lung (Figure 5-11). Here the Po_2 at the apex is some 40 mm Hg higher than at the base of the lung. However, the major share of the blood leaving the lung comes from the lower zones, where the Po_2 is low. This has the result of depressing the arterial Po_2. By contrast, the expired alveolar gas comes more uniformly from apex and base because the differences of ventilation are much less than those for blood flow (Figure 5-8). By the same reasoning, the arterial Pco_2 will be elevated because it is higher at the base of the lung than at the apex (Figure 5-10).

An additional reason that uneven ventilation and blood flow depress the arterial Po_2 is shown in Figure 5-12. This depicts three groups of alveoli with low, normal, and high ventilation-perfusion ratios. The O_2 concentrations of the effluent blood are 16, 19.5, and 20 ml 100 ml^{-1}, respectively. As a result, the units with the high

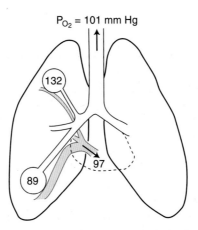

P_{O_2} = 101 mm Hg

132

97

89

Figure 5-11. Depression of the arterial Po_2 by ventilation-perfusion inequality. In this diagram of the upright lung, only two groups of alveoli are shown, one at the apex and another at the base. The relative sizes of the airways and blood vessels indicate their relative ventilations and blood flows. Because most of the blood comes from the poorly oxygenated base, depression of the blood Po_2 is inevitable.

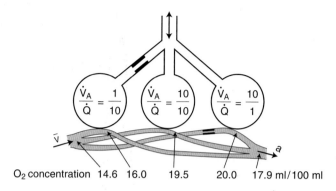

O₂ concentration 14.6 16.0   19.5   20.0   17.9 ml/100 ml

Figure 5-12. Additional reason for the depression of arterial P_{O_2} by mismatching of ventilation and blood flow. The lung units with a high ventilation-perfusion ratio add relatively little oxygen to the blood, compared with the decrement caused by alveoli with a low ventilation-perfusion ratio.

ventilation-perfusion ratio add relatively little oxygen to the blood, compared with the decrement caused by the alveoli with the low ventilation-perfusion ratio. Thus, the mixed capillary blood has a lower O_2 concentration than that from units with a normal ventilation-perfusion ratio. This can be explained by the nonlinear shape of the oxygen dissociation curve, which means that although units with a high ventilation-perfusion ratio have a relatively high P_{O_2}, this does not increase the oxygen concentration of their blood very much. This additional reason for the depression of P_{O_2} does not apply to the elevation of the P_{CO_2} because the CO_2 dissociation curve is almost linear in the working range.

The net result of these mechanisms is a depression of the arterial P_{O_2} below that of the mixed alveolar P_{O_2}—the so-called alveolar-arterial O_2 difference. In the normal upright lung, this difference is of trivial magnitude, being only about 4 mm Hg due to ventilation-perfusion inequality. Its development is described here only to illustrate how uneven ventilation and blood flow must result in depression of the arterial P_{O_2}. In lung disease, the lowering of arterial P_{O_2} by this mechanism can be extreme.

► Distributions of Ventilation-Perfusion Ratios

It is possible to obtain information about the distribution of ventilation-perfusion ratios in patients with lung disease by infusing into a peripheral vein a mixture of dissolved inert gases having a range of solubilities and then measuring the concentrations of the gases in arterial blood and expired gas. The details of this technique are too complex to be described here, and it is used for research purposes rather than in the pulmonary function laboratory. The technique returns a distribution of ventilation and blood flow plotted against ventilation-perfusion ratio with 50 compartments equally spaced on a log scale.

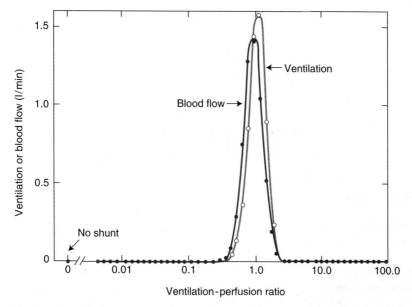

Figure 5-13. Distribution of ventilation-perfusion ratios in a young normal subject. Note the narrow dispersion and absence of shunt.

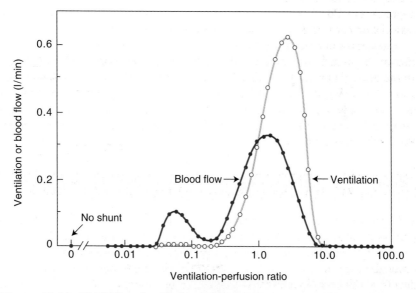

Figure 5-14. Distribution of ventilation-perfusion ratios in a patient with chronic bronchitis and emphysema. Note particularly the blood flow to lung units with very low ventilation-perfusion ratios. Compare Figure 5-13.

Figure 5-13 shows a typical result from a young normal subject. Note that all the ventilation and blood flow goes to compartments close to the normal ventilation-perfusion ratio of about 1.0, and, in particular, there is no blood flow to the unventilated compartment (shunt). The distributions in patients with lung disease are often very different. An example from a patient with chronic bronchitis and emphysema is shown in Figure 5-14. Note that although much of the ventilation and blood flow goes to compartments with ventilation-perfusion ratios near normal, considerable blood flow is going to compartments with ventilation-perfusion ratios of between 0.03 and 0.3. Blood from these units will be poorly oxygenated and will depress the arterial Po_2. There is also excessive ventilation to lung units with ventilation-perfusion ratios up to 10. These units are inefficient at eliminating CO_2. This particular patient had arterial hypoxemia but a normal arterial Pco_2 (see below). Other patterns are seen in other types of lung disease.

► Ventilation-Perfusion Inequality as a Cause of CO_2 Retention

Imagine a lung that is uniformly ventilated and perfused and that is transferring normal amounts of O_2 and CO_2. Suppose that in some magical way, the matching of ventilation and blood flow is suddenly disturbed while everything else remains unchanged. What happens to gas exchange? It transpires that the effect of this "pure" ventilation-perfusion inequality (that is, everything else held constant) is to reduce *both* the O_2 uptake and CO_2 output of the lung. In other words, the lung becomes less efficient as a gas exchanger for both gases. Hence, mismatching ventilation and blood flow must cause both hypoxemia and hypercapnia (CO_2 retention), other things being equal.

Ventilation-Perfusion Inequality

- The ventilation-perfusion ratio ($\dot{V}_A / \dot{Q}$) determines the gas exchange in any single lung unit
- Regional differences of $\dot{V}_A / \dot{Q}$ in the upright human lung cause a pattern of regional gas exchange
- $\dot{V}_A / \dot{Q}$ inequality impairs the uptake or elimination of all gases by the lung
- Although the elimination of CO_2 is impaired by $\dot{V}_A / \dot{Q}$ inequality, this can be corrected by increasing the ventilation to the alveoli
- By contrast, the hypoxemia resulting from $\dot{V}_A / \dot{Q}$ inequality cannot be eliminated by increases in ventilation
- The different behavior of the two gases results from the different shapes of their dissociation curves

However, in practice, patients with undoubted ventilation-perfusion inequality often have a normal arterial P_{CO_2}. The reason for this is that whenever the chemoreceptors sense a rising P_{CO_2}, there is an increase in ventilatory drive (Chapter 8). The consequent increase in ventilation to the alveoli is usually effective in returning the arterial P_{CO_2} to normal. However, such patients can only maintain a normal P_{CO_2} at the expense of this increased ventilation to their alveoli; the ventilation in excess of what they would normally require is sometimes referred to as *wasted ventilation* and is necessary because the lung units with abnormally high ventilation-perfusion ratios are inefficient at eliminating CO_2. Such units are said to constitute an *alveolar dead space*.

While the increase in ventilation to a lung with ventilation-perfusion inequality is usually effective at reducing the arterial P_{CO_2}, it is much less effective at increasing the arterial P_{O_2}. The reason for the different behavior of the two gases lies in the shapes of the CO_2 and O_2 dissociation curves (Chapter 6). The CO_2 dissociation curve is almost straight in the physiological range, with the result that an increase in ventilation will raise the CO_2 output of lung units with both high and low ventilation-perfusion ratios. By contrast, the almost flat top of the O_2 dissociation curve means that only units with moderately low ventilation-perfusion ratios will benefit appreciably from the increased ventilation. Those units that are very high on the dissociation curve (high ventilation-perfusion ratio) increase the O_2 concentration of their effluent blood very little (Figure 5-12). Those units that have a very low ventilation-perfusion ratio continue to put out blood with an O_2 concentration close to that of mixed venous blood. The net result is that the mixed arterial P_{O_2} rises only modestly, and some hypoxemia always remains.

▶ Measurement of Ventilation-Perfusion Inequality

How can we assess the amount of ventilation-perfusion inequality in diseased lungs? Radioactive gases can be used to define topographical differences in ventilation and blood flow in the normal upright lung (Figures 2-7 and 4-7), but in most patients large amounts of inequality exist between closely adjacent units, and this cannot be distinguished by counters over the chest. In practice, we turn to indices based on the resulting impairment of gas exchange.[†]

One useful measurement is the *alveolar-arterial* P_{O_2} *difference*, obtained by subtracting the arterial P_{O_2} from the so-called ideal alveolar P_{O_2}. The latter

---

[†]For more details of this difficult subject, see JB West, *Pulmonary Pathophysiology: The Essentials*, 7th ed. (Baltimore, MD: Lippincott Williams & Wilkins, 2007).

is the P_{O_2} that the lung *would* have if there were no ventilation-perfusion inequality, and it was exchanging gas at the same respiratory exchange ratio as the real lung. It is derived from the alveolar gas equation:

$$P_{A_{O_2}} = P_{I_{O_2}} - \frac{P_{A_{CO_2}}}{R} + F$$

The arterial P_{CO_2} is used for the alveolar value.

An example will clarify this. Suppose a patient who is breathing air at sea level has an arterial P_{O_2} of 50 mm Hg, an arterial P_{CO_2} of 60 mm Hg, and a respiratory exchange ratio of 0.8. Could the arterial hypoxemia be explained by hypoventilation?

From the alveolar gas equation, the ideal alveolar P_{O_2} is given by

$$P_{A_{O_2}} = 149 - \frac{60}{0.8} + F = 7.4 \text{ mm Hg}$$

where the inspired P_{O_2} is 149 mm Hg and we ignore the small factor F. Thus, the alveolar-arterial P_{O_2} difference is approximately $(74 - 50) = 24$ mm Hg. This is abnormally high and indicates that there is ventilation-perfusion inequality.

Additional information on the measurement of ventilation-perfusion inequality can be found in Chapter 10.

KEY CONCEPTS

1. The four causes of hypoxemia are hypoventilation, diffusion limitation, shunt, and ventilation-perfusion inequality.
2. The two causes of hypercapnia, or CO_2 retention, are hypoventilation and ventilation-perfusion inequality.
3. Shunt is the only cause of hypoxemia in which the arterial P_{O_2} does not rise to the expected level when a patient is given 100% O_2 to breathe.
4. The ventilation-perfusion ratio determines the P_{O_2} and P_{CO_2} in any lung unit. Because the ratio is high at the top of the lung, P_{O_2} is high there and the P_{CO_2} is low.
5. Ventilation-perfusion inequality reduces the gas exchange efficiency of the lung for all gases. However, many patients with ventilation-perfusion inequality have a normal arterial P_{CO_2} because they increase the ventilation to their alveoli. By contrast, the arterial P_{O_2} is always low. The different behavior of the two gases is attributable to the different shapes of the two dissociation curves.
6. The alveolar-arterial P_{O_2} difference is a useful measure of ventilation-perfusion inequality. The alveolar P_{O_2} is calculated from the alveolar gas equation using the arterial P_{CO_2}.

QUESTIONS

For each question, choose the one best answer.

1. A climber reaches an altitude of 4,500 m (14,800 ft) where the barometric pressure is 447 mm Hg. The P_{O_2} of moist inspired gas (in mm Hg) is
   A. 47
   B. 63
   C. 75
   D. 84
   E. 98

2. A man with normal lungs and an arterial P_{CO_2} of 40 mm Hg takes an overdose of barbiturate that halves his alveolar ventilation but does not change his CO_2 output. If his respiratory exchange ratio is 0.8, what will be his arterial P_{O_2} (in mm Hg), approximately?
   A. 40
   B. 50
   C. 60
   D. 70
   E. 80

3. In the situation described in Question 2, how much does the inspired O_2 concentration (%) have to be raised to return the arterial P_{O_2} to its original level?
   A. 7
   B. 11
   C. 15
   D. 19
   E. 23

4. A patient with normal lungs but a right-to-left shunt is found at catheterization to have oxygen concentrations in his arterial and mixed venous blood of 18 and 14 ml·100 ml⁻¹, respectively. If the O_2 concentration of the blood leaving the pulmonary capillaries is calculated to be 20 ml · 100 ml⁻¹, what is his shunt as a percentage of his cardiac output?
   A. 23
   B. 33
   C. 43
   D. 53
   E. 63

5. If a climber on the summit of Mt. Everest (barometric pressure 247 mm Hg) maintains an alveolar P_{O_2} of 34 mm Hg and is in a steady state ($R \leq 1$), his alveolar P_{CO_2} (in mm Hg) cannot be any higher than
   A. 5
   B. 8
   C. 10
   D. 12
   E. 15

6. A patient with severe chronic obstructive pulmonary disease, which causes marked ventilation-perfusion inequality, has an arterial Po_2 of 50 mm Hg and an arterial Pco_2 of 40 mm Hg. The Pco_2 is normal despite the hypoxemia because

   A. Ventilation-perfusion inequality does not interfere with CO_2 elimination.
   B. Much of the CO_2 is carried as bicarbonate.
   C. The formation of carbonic acid is accelerated by carbonic anhydrase.
   D. CO_2 diffuses much faster through tissue than O_2.
   E. The O_2 and CO_2 dissociation curves have different shapes.

7. The apex of the upright human lung compared with the base has

   A. A higher Po_2.
   B. A higher ventilation.
   C. A lower pH in end-capillary blood.
   D. A higher blood flow.
   E. Smaller alveoli.

8. If the ventilation-perfusion ratio of a lung unit is decreased by partial bronchial obstruction while the rest of the lung is unaltered, the affected lung unit will show

   A. Increased alveolar Po_2.
   B. Decreased alveolar Pco_2.
   C. No change in alveolar PN_2.
   D. A rise in pH of end-capillary blood.
   E. A fall in oxygen uptake.

9. A patient with lung disease who is breathing air has an arterial Po_2 and Pco_2 of 49 and 48 mm Hg, respectively, and a respiratory exchange ratio of 0.8. The approximate alveolar-arterial difference for Po_2 (in mm Hg) is

   A. 10
   B. 20
   C. 30
   D. 40
   E. 50

Gas Transport by the Blood

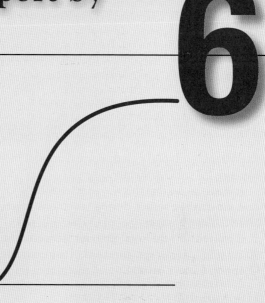

6

▶ **HOW GASES ARE MOVED TO AND FROM THE PERIPHERAL TISSUES**

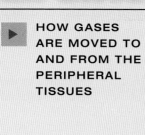

We now consider the carriage of the respiratory gases, oxygen and carbon dioxide, by the blood. First, we look at the oxygen dissociation curve, including the factors that affect the oxygen affinity of hemoglobin. Then we turn to carbon dioxide, which is carried in the blood in three forms. Next, we consider the acid-base status of the blood and the four principal abnormalities: respiratory acidosis and alkalosis, and metabolic acidosis and alkalosis. Finally, we briefly look at gas exchange in peripheral tissues.

▶ Oxygen

O_2 is carried in the blood in two forms: dissolved and combined with hemoglobin.

Dissolved O_2

This obeys Henry's law, that is, the amount dissolved is proportional to the partial pressure (Figure 6-1). For each mm Hg of Po_2, there is 0.003 ml $O_2 \cdot 100$ ml^{-1} of blood. Thus, normal arterial blood with a Po_2 of 100 mm Hg contains 0.3 ml $O_2 \cdot 100$ ml^{-1}.

It is easy to see that this way of transporting O_2 must be inadequate. Suppose that the cardiac output during strenuous exercise is 30 liters·min^{-1}. Because arterial blood contains 0.3 ml $O_2 \cdot 100$ ml^{-1} blood (that is, 3 ml $O_2 \cdot$liter^{-1} blood) as dissolved O_2, the total amount delivered to the tissues is only 30 × 3 = 90 ml·min^{-1}. However, the tissue requirements may be as high as 3000 ml $O_2 \cdot$min^{-1}. Clearly, an additional method of transporting O_2 is required.

Hemoglobin

Heme is an iron-porphyrin compound; this is joined to the protein globin, which consists of four polypeptide chains. The chains are of two types, alpha and beta, and differences in their amino acid sequences give rise to various types of human hemoglobin. Normal adult hemoglobin is known as A. Hemoglobin F (fetal)

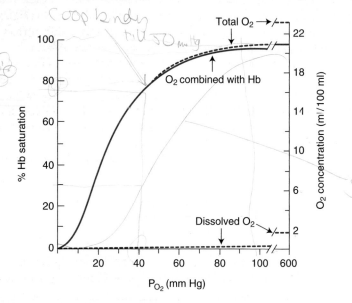

Figure 6-1. O_2 dissociation curve (*solid line*) for pH 7.4, Pco_2 40 mm Hg, and 37°C. The total blood O_2 concentration is also shown for a hemoglobin concentration of 15 g·100 ml^{-1} of blood.

makes up part of the hemoglobin of the newborn infant and is gradually replaced over the first year or so of postnatal life. Hemoglobin S (sickle) has valine instead of glutamic acid in the beta chains. This results in a reduced O_2 affinity and a shift in the dissociation curve to the right, but, more important, the deoxygenated form is poorly soluble and crystallizes within the red cell. As a consequence, the cell shape changes from biconcave to crescent or sickle shaped with increased fragility and a tendency to thrombus formation. Many other varieties of hemoglobin have now been described, some with bizarre O_2 affinities. For more information about hemoglobin, consult a textbook of biochemistry.

Normal hemoglobin A can have its ferrous ion oxidized to the ferric form by various drugs and chemicals, including nitrites, sulfonamides, and acetanilid. This ferric form is known as methemoglobin. There is a congenital cause in which the enzyme methemoglobin reductase is deficient within the red blood cell. Another abnormal form is sulfhemoglobin. These compounds are not useful for O_2 carriage.

O_2 Dissociation Curve

O_2 forms an easily reversible combination with hemoglobin (Hb) to give oxyhemoglobin: $O_2 + Hb \rightleftharpoons HbO_2$. Suppose we take a number of glass containers (tonometers), each containing a small volume of blood, and add gas with various concentrations of O_2. After allowing time for the gas and blood to reach equilibrium, we measure the Po_2 of the gas and the O_2 concentration of the blood. Knowing that 0.003 ml O_2 will be dissolved in each 100 ml of blood·mm^{-1} Hg Po_2, we can calculate the O_2 combined with Hb (Figure 6-1). Note that the amount of O_2 carried by the Hb increases rapidly up to a Po_2 of about 50 mm Hg, but above that, the curve becomes much flatter.

The maximum amount of O_2 that can be combined with Hb is called the *O_2 capacity*. This is when all the available binding sites are occupied by O_2. It can be measured by exposing the blood to a very high Po_2 (say 600 mm Hg) and subtracting the dissolved O_2. One gram of pure Hb can combine with 1.39* ml O_2, and because normal blood has about 15 g of Hb·100 ml^{-1}, the O_2 capacity is about 20.8 ml O_2·100 ml^{-1} of blood.

The *O_2 saturation* of Hb is the percentage of the available binding sites that have O_2 attached and is given by

$$\frac{O_2 \text{ combined with Hb}}{O_2 \text{ capacity}} \times 100$$

The O_2 saturation of arterial blood with Po_2 of 100 mm Hg is about 97.5%, whereas that of mixed venous blood with a Po_2 of 40 mm Hg is about 75%.

---

*Some measurements give 1.34 or 1.36 ml. The reason is that under the normal conditions of the body, some of the hemoglobin is in forms such as methemoglobin that cannot combine with O_2.

Usually 15 g

9/16

layer Hb
layer O cap
correct

20.8 × 10
15

The change in Hb from the fully oxygenated state to its deoxygenated state is accompanied by a conformational change in the molecule. The oxygenated form is the R (relaxed) state, whereas the deoxy form is the T (tense) state. It is important to grasp the relationships among P_{O_2}, O_2 saturation, and O_2 concentration (Figure 6-2). For example, suppose a severely anemic patient with an Hb concentration of only 10 g·100 ml^{-1} of blood has normal lungs and an arterial P_{O_2} of 100 mm Hg. This patient's O_2 capacity will be 20.8 × 10/15 = 13.9 ml·100 ml^{-1}. The patient's O_2 saturation will be 97.5% (at normal pH, P_{CO_2}, and temperature), but the O_2 combined with Hb will be only 13.5 ml 100 ml^{-1}. Dissolved O_2 will contribute 0.3 ml, giving a total O_2 concentration of 13.8·ml 100 ml^{-1} of blood. In general, the oxygen concentration of blood (in ml O_2·100 ml^{-1} blood) is given by

$$\left(1.39 \times \text{Hb} \times \frac{\text{Sat}}{100}\right) + 0.003\,P_{O_2}$$

where Hb is the hemoglobin concentration in g·100 ml^{-1}, Sat is the percentage saturation of the hemoglobin, and P_{O_2} is in mm Hg.

The curved shape of the O_2 dissociation curve has several physiological advantages. The flat upper portion means that even if the P_{O_2} in alveolar gas falls somewhat, loading of O_2 will be little affected. In addition, as the red cell takes up O_2 along the pulmonary capillary (Figure 3-3), a large partial pressure difference between alveolar gas and blood continues to exist when most of the O_2 has been transferred. As a result, the diffusion process is hastened. The steep lower part of the dissociation curve means that the peripheral tissues

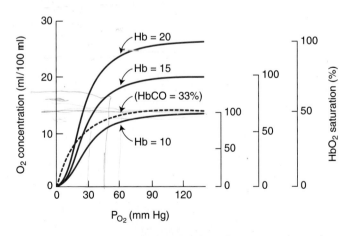

Figure 6-2. Effects of anemia and polycythemia on O_2 concentration and saturation. In addition, the *broken line* shows the O_2 dissociation curve when one-third of the normal hemoglobin is bound to CO. Note that the curve is then shifted to the left.

can withdraw large amounts of O_2 for only a small drop in capillary Po_2. This maintenance of blood Po_2 assists the diffusion of O_2 into the tissue cells.

Because reduced Hb is purple, a low arterial O_2 saturation causes *cyanosis*. However, this is not a reliable sign of mild desaturation because its recognition depends on so many variables, such as lighting conditions and skin pigmentation. Because it is the amount of reduced Hb that is important, cyanosis is often marked when polycythemia is present but is difficult to detect in anemic patients.

The O_2 dissociation curve is shifted to the right, that is, the O_2 affinity of Hb is reduced, by an increase in H^+ concentration, Pco_2, temperature, and the concentration of 2,3-diphosphoglycerate in the red cells (Figure 6-3). Opposite changes shift it to the left. Most of the effect of Pco_2, which is known as the *Bohr effect*, can be attributed to its action on H^+ concentration. A rightward shift means more unloading of O_2 at a given Po_2 in a tissue capillary. A simple way to remember these shifts is that an exercising muscle is acid, hypercarbic, and hot, and it benefits from increased unloading of O_2 from its capillaries.

The environment of the Hb within the red cell also affects the O_2 dissociation curve. An increase in 2,3-diphosphoglycerate (DPG), which is an end product of red cell metabolism, shifts the curve to the right. An increase

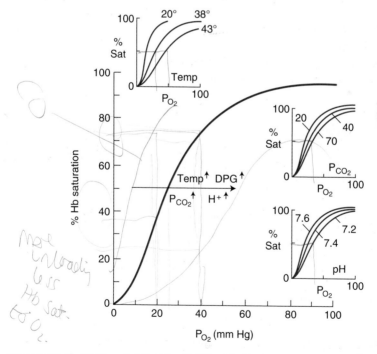

Figure 6-3. Rightward shift of the O_2 dissociation curve by increase of H^+, Pco_2, temperature, and 2,3-diphosphoglycerate (DPG).

in concentration of this material occurs in chronic hypoxia, for example, at high altitude or in the presence of chronic lung disease. As a result, the unloading of O_2 to peripheral tissues is assisted. By contrast, stored blood in a blood bank may be depleted of 2,3-DPG, and unloading of O_2 is therefore impaired. A useful measure of the position of the dissociation curve is the Po_2 for 50% O_2 saturation. This is known as the P_{50}. The normal value for human blood is about 27 mm Hg.

Oxygen Dissociation Curve

- Useful "anchor" points: Po_2 40, So_2 75%; Po_2 100, So_2 97%
- Curve is right-shifted by increases in temperature, Pco_2, H^+, and 2,3-DPG
- Small addition of CO to blood causes a left shift

Carbon monoxide interferes with the O_2 transport function of blood by combining with Hb to form carboxyhemoglobin (COHb). CO has about 240 times the affinity of O_2 for Hb; this means that CO will combine with the same amount of Hb as O_2 when the CO partial pressure is 240 times lower. In fact, the CO dissociation curve is almost identical in shape to the O_2 dissociation curve of Figure 6-3, except that the P_{CO} axis is greatly compressed. For example, at a P_{CO} of 0.16 mm Hg, about 75% of the Hb is combined with CO as COHb. For this reason, small amounts of CO can tie up a large proportion of the Hb in the blood, thus making it unavailable for O_2 carriage. If this happens, the Hb concentration and Po_2 of blood may be normal, but its O_2 concentration is grossly reduced. The presence of COHb also shifts the O_2 dissociation curve to the left (Figure 6-2), thus interfering with the unloading of O_2. This is an additional feature of the toxicity of CO.

▶ Carbon Dioxide

CO_2 Carriage

CO_2 is carried in the blood in three forms: dissolved, as bicarbonate, and in combination with proteins as carbamino compounds (Figure 6-4).

1. *Dissolved CO_2*, like O_2, obeys Henry's law, but CO_2 is about 20 times more soluble than O_2, its solubility being 0.067 ml·dl⁻¹·mm Hg⁻¹. As a result, dissolved CO_2 plays a significant role in its carriage in that about 10% of the gas that is evolved into the lung from the blood is in the dissolved form (Figure 6-4).

2. *Bicarbonate* is formed in blood by the following sequence:

$$CO_2 + H_2O \overset{CA}{\rightleftharpoons} H_2CO_3 \rightleftharpoons H^+ + HCO_3^-$$

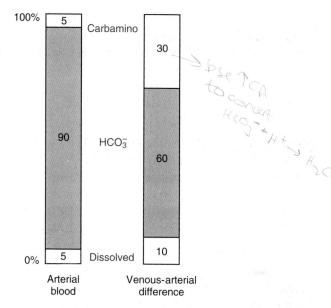

Figure 6-4. The *first column* shows the proportions of the total CO_2 concentration in arterial blood. The *second column* shows the proportions that make up the venous-arterial difference.

The first reaction is very slow in plasma but fast within the red blood cell because of the presence there of the enzyme *carbonic anhydrase* (CA). The second reaction, ionic dissociation of carbonic acid, is fast without an enzyme. When the concentration of these ions rises within the red cell, HCO_3^- diffuses out, but H^+ cannot easily do this because the cell membrane is relatively impermeable to cations. Thus, to maintain electrical neutrality, Cl^- ions move into the cell from the plasma, the so-called *chloride shift* (Figure 6-5). The movement of chloride is in accordance with the Gibbs-Donnan equilibrium.

Some of the H^+ ions liberated are bound to reduced hemoglobin:

$$H^+ + HbO_2 \rightleftharpoons H^+ \cdot Hb + O_2$$

This occurs because reduced Hb is less acid (that is, a better proton acceptor) than the oxygenated form. Thus, the presence of reduced Hb in the peripheral blood helps with the loading of CO_2, whereas the oxygenation that occurs in the pulmonary capillary assists in the unloading. The fact that deoxygenation of the blood increases its ability to carry CO_2 is known as the *Haldane effect*.

These events associated with the uptake of CO_2 by blood increase the osmolar content of the red cell, and, consequently, water enters the cell, thus increasing its volume. When the cells pass through the lung, they shrink a little.

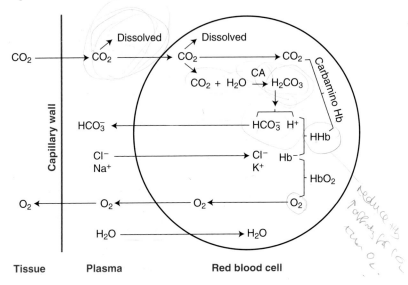

Figure 6-5. Scheme of the uptake of CO_2 and liberation of O_2 in systemic capillaries. Exactly opposite events occur in the pulmonary capillaries.

3. *Carbamino compounds* are formed by the combination of CO_2 with terminal amine groups in blood proteins. The most important protein is the globin of hemoglobin: $Hb \cdot NH_2 + CO_2 \rightleftharpoons Hb \cdot NH \cdot COOH$, giving carbaminohemoglobin. This reaction occurs rapidly without an enzyme, and reduced Hb can bind more CO_2 as carbaminohemoglobin than HbO_2. Thus, again, unloading of O_2 in peripheral capillaries facilitates the loading of CO_2, whereas oxygenation has the opposite effect.

The relative contributions of the various forms of CO_2 in blood to the total CO_2 concentration are summarized in Figure 6-4. Note that the great bulk of the CO_2 is in the form of bicarbonate. The amount dissolved is small, as is that in the form of carbaminohemoglobin. However, these proportions do not reflect the changes that take place when CO_2 is loaded or unloaded by the blood. Of the total venous-arterial difference, about 60% is attributable to HCO_3^-, 30% to carbamino compounds, and 10% to dissolved CO_2.

CO_2 Dissociation Curve

The relationship between the Pco_2 and the total CO_2 concentration of blood is shown in Figure 6-6. By analogy with O_2, this is often (though loosely) referred to as the CO_2 dissociation curve, and it is much more linear than is the O_2 dissociation curve (Figure 6-1). Note also that the lower the saturation of Hb with O_2, the larger the CO_2 concentration for a given Pco_2. As we have seen, this *Haldane effect* can be explained by the better ability of reduced Hb to mop up the H^+ ions produced when carbonic acid dissociates, and the

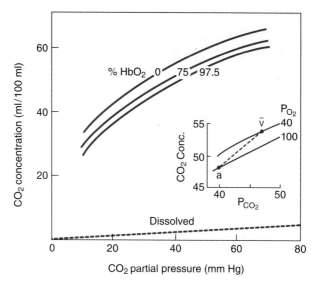

Figure 6-6. CO_2 dissociation curves for blood of different O_2 saturations. Note that oxygenated blood carries less CO_2 for the same Pco_2. The *inset* shows the "physiological" curve between arterial and mixed venous blood.

greater facility of reduced Hb to form carbaminohemoglobin. Figure 6-7 shows that the CO_2 dissociation curve is considerably steeper than that for O_2. For example, in the range of 40 to 50 mm Hg, the CO_2 concentration changes by about 4.7, compared with an O_2 concentration of only about 1.7 ml/100 ml. This is why the Po_2 difference between arterial and mixed venous blood is large (typically about 60 mm Hg) but the Pco_2 difference is small (about 5 mm Hg).

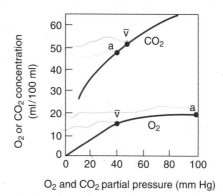

Figure 6-7. Typical O_2 and CO_2 dissociation curves plotted with the same scales. Note that the CO_2 curve is much steeper. *a* and *v̄* refer to arterial and mixed venous blood, respectively.

Carbon Dioxide Dissociation Curve

- CO_2 is carried as dissolved, bicarbonate, and carbamino
- CO_2 curve is steeper and more linear than the O_2 curve
- CO_2 curve is right-shifted by increases in So_2

▶ Acid-Base Status

The transport of CO_2 has a profound effect on the acid-base status of the blood and the body as a whole. The lung excretes over 10,000 mEq of carbonic acid per day, compared with less than 100 mEq of fixed acids by the kidney. Therefore, by altering alveolar ventilation and thus the elimination of CO_2, the body has great control over its acid-base balance. This subject will be treated only briefly here because it overlaps the area of renal physiology.

The pH resulting from the solution of CO_2 in blood and the consequent dissociation of carbonic acid is given by the Henderson-Hasselbalch equation. It is derived as follows. In the equation

$$H_2CO_3 \rightleftharpoons H^+ + HCO_3^-$$

the law of the mass action gives the dissociation constant of carbonic acid K'_A as

$$\frac{(H^+) \times (HCO_3^-)}{(H_2CO_3)}$$

Because the concentration of carbonic acid is proportional to the concentration of dissolved carbon dioxide, we can change the constant and write

$$K_A = \frac{(H^+) \times (HCO_3^-)}{(CO_2)}$$

Taking logarithms,

$$\log K_A = \log(H^+) + \log\frac{(HCO_3^-)}{(CO_2)}$$

whence

$$-\log(H^+) = -\log K_A + \log\frac{(HCO_3^-)}{(CO_2)}$$

Because pH is the negative logarithm,

$$pH = pK_A + \log\frac{(HCO_3^-)}{(CO_2)}$$

Because CO_2 obeys Henry's law, the CO_2 concentration (in $mmol\cdot l^{-1}$) can be replaced by ($Pco_2 \times 0.03$). The equation then becomes

$$pH = pK_A + \log\frac{(HCO_3^-)}{0.03 Pco_2}$$

The value of pK_A is 6.1, and the normal HCO_3^- concentration in arterial blood is 24 $mmol\cdot l^{-1}$. Substituting gives

$$
\begin{aligned}
pH &= 6.1 + \log\frac{24}{0.03 \times 40} \\
&= 6.1 + \log 20 \\
&= 6.1 + 1.3
\end{aligned}
$$

Therefore,

$$pH = 7.4$$

Note that as long as the ratio of bicarbonate concentration to ($Pco_2 \times 0.03$) remains equal to 20, the pH will remain at 7.4. The bicarbonate concentration is determined chiefly by the kidney and the Pco_2 by the lung.

The relationships among pH, Pco_2, and HCO_3^- are conveniently shown on a Davenport diagram (Figure 6-8). The two axes show HCO_3^- and pH, and lines of equal Pco_2 sweep across the diagram. Normal plasma is represented by point A. The line CAB shows the relationship between HCO_3^- and pH as carbonic acid is added to whole blood, that is, it is part of the titration curve for blood and is called the *buffer line*. Also, the slope of this line is steeper than that measured in plasma separated from blood because of the presence of hemoglobin, which has an additional buffering action. The slope of the line measured on whole blood *in vitro* is usually a little different from that found in a patient because of the buffering action of the interstitial fluid and other body tissues.

If the plasma bicarbonate concentration is altered by the kidney, the buffer line is displaced. An increase in bicarbonate concentration displaces the buffer line upward, as shown, for example, by line DE in Figure 6-8. In this case, a *base excess* exists and is given by the vertical distance between the two buffer lines DE and BAC. By contrast, a reduced bicarbonate concentration displaces the buffer line downward (line GF), and there is now a negative base excess, or *base deficit*.

A

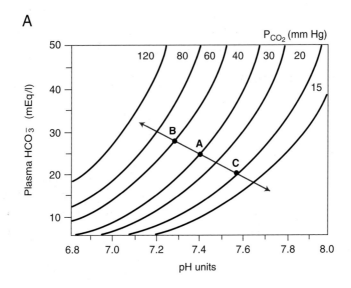

B

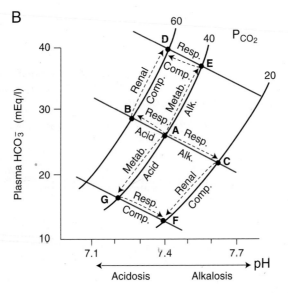

Figure 6-8. Davenport diagram showing the relationships among HCO_3^-, pH, and P_{CO_2}. **A** shows the normal buffer line BAC. **B** shows the changes occurring in respiratory and metabolic acidosis and alkalosis (see text). The vertical distance between the buffer lines DE and BAC is the base excess, and that between lines GF and BAC is the base deficit (or negative base excess).

The ratio of bicarbonate to P_{CO_2} can be disturbed in four ways: both P_{CO_2} and bicarbonate can be raised or lowered. Each of these four disturbances gives rise to a characteristic acid-base change.

Respiratory Acidosis

Respiratory acidosis is caused by an increase in P_{CO_2}, which reduces the HCO_3^- / P_{CO_2} ratio and thus depresses the pH. This corresponds to a movement from A to B in Figure 6-8. Whenever the P_{CO_2} rises, the bicarbonate must also increase to some extent because of dissociation of the carbonic acid produced. This is reflected by the left upward slope of the blood buffer line in Figure 6-8. However, the ratio HCO_3^- / P_{CO_2} falls. CO_2 retention can be caused by hypoventilation or ventilation-perfusion inequality.

If respiratory acidosis persists, the kidney responds by conserving HCO_3^-. It is prompted to do this by the increased P_{CO_2} in the renal tubular cells, which then excrete a more acid urine by secreting H^+ ions. The H^+ ions are excreted as $H_2PO_4^-$ or NH_4^+; the HCO_3^- ions are reabsorbed. The resulting increase in plasma HCO_3^- then moves the HCO_3^- / P_{CO_2} ratio back up toward its normal level. This corresponds to the movement from B to D along the line $P_{CO_2} = 60$ mm Hg in Figure 6-8 and is known as *compensated respiratory acidosis*. Typical events would be

$$pH = 6.1 + \log \frac{24}{0.03 \times 40} = 6.1 + \log 20 = 7.4 \quad \text{(Normal)}$$

$$pH = 6.1 + \log \frac{28}{0.03 \times 60} = 6.1 + \log 15.6 = 7.29 \quad \text{(Respiratory acidosis)}$$

$$pH = 6.1 + \log \frac{33}{0.03 \times 60} = 6.1 + \log 18.3 = 7.36 \text{ (Compensated respiratory acidosis)}$$

The renal compensation is typically not complete, and so the pH does not fully return to its normal level of 7.4. The extent of the renal compensation can be determined from the *base excess*, that is, the vertical distance between the buffer lines BA and DE.

Respiratory Alkalosis

This is caused by a decrease in P_{CO_2}, which increases the HCO_3^- / P_{CO_2} ratio and thus elevates the pH (movement from A to C in Figure 6-8). A decrease in P_{CO_2} is caused by hyperventilation, for example, at high altitude (see Chapter 9). Renal compensation occurs by an increased excretion of bicarbonate, thus returning the HCO_3^- / P_{CO_2} ratio back toward normal (C to F along the line P_{CO_2} = 20 mm Hg). After a prolonged stay at high altitude, the renal compensation may be nearly complete. There is a negative base excess, or a *base deficit*.

Four Types of Acid-Base Disturbances		
$$pH = pK + \log \frac{HCO_3^-}{0.03\ P_{CO_2}}$$		
	Primary	**Compensation**
Acidosis		
Respiratory	$P_{CO_2}\uparrow$	$HCO_3^-\uparrow$
Metabolic	$HCO_3^-\downarrow$	$P_{CO_2}\downarrow$
Alkalosis		
Respiratory	$P_{CO_2}\downarrow$	$HCO_3^-\downarrow$
Metabolic	$HCO_3^-\uparrow$	Often none

Metabolic Acidosis

In this context, "metabolic" means a primary change in HCO_3^-, that is, the numerator of the Henderson-Hasselbalch equation. In metabolic acidosis, the ratio of HCO_3^- to P_{CO_2} falls, thus depressing the pH. The HCO_3^- may be lowered by the accumulation of acids in the blood, as in uncontrolled diabetes mellitus, or after tissue hypoxia, which releases lactic acid. The corresponding change in Figure 6-8 is a movement from A toward G.

In this instance, respiratory compensation occurs by an increase in ventilation that lowers the P_{CO_2} and raises the depressed HCO_3^-/P_{CO_2} ratio. The stimulus to raise the ventilation is chiefly the action of H^+ ions on the peripheral chemoreceptors (Chapter 8). In Figure 6-8, the point moves in the direction G to F (although not as far as F). There is a base deficit or negative base excess.

Metabolic Alkalosis

Here an increase in HCO_3^- raises the HCO_3^-/P_{CO_2} ratio and, thus, the pH. Excessive ingestion of alkalis and loss of acid gastric secretion by vomiting are causes. In Figure 6-8, the movement is in the direction A to E. Some respiratory compensation sometimes occurs by a reduction in alveolar ventilation that raises the P_{CO_2}. Point E then moves in the direction of D (although not all the way). However, respiratory compensation in metabolic alkalosis is often small and may be absent. Base excess is increased.

Note that mixed respiratory and metabolic disturbances often occur, and it may then be difficult to unravel the sequence of events.

▶ Blood-Tissue Gas Exchange

O_2 and CO_2 move between the systemic capillary blood and the tissue cells by simple diffusion, just as they move between the capillary blood and alveolar gas in the lung. We saw in Chapter 3 that the rate of transfer of gas through a tissue sheet is proportional to the tissue area and the difference in gas partial pressure between the two sides, and inversely proportional to the thickness. The thickness of the blood-gas barrier is less than 0.5 μm, but the distance between open capillaries in resting muscle is on the order of 50 μm. During exercise, when the O_2 consumption of the muscle increases, additional capillaries open up, thus reducing the diffusion distance and increasing the area for diffusion. Because CO_2 diffuses about 20 times faster than O_2 through tissue (Figure 3-1), elimination of CO_2 is much less of a problem than is O_2 delivery.

The way in which the Po_2 falls in tissue between adjacent open capillaries is shown schematically in Figure 6-9. As the O_2 diffuses away from the capillary, it is consumed by tissue, and the Po_2 falls. In A, the balance between O_2 consumption and delivery (determined by the capillary Po_2 and the intercapillary distance) results in an adequate Po_2 in all the tissue. In B, the intercapillary distance or the O_2 consumption has been increased until the Po_2 at one point in the tissue falls to zero. This is referred to as a *critical* situation. In C, there is an anoxic region where aerobic (that is, O_2 utilizing) metabolism is impossible. Under these conditions, the tissue may turn to anaerobic glycolysis with the formation of lactic acid.

There is evidence that much of the fall of Po_2 in peripheral tissues occurs in the immediate vicinity of the capillary wall and that the Po_2 in muscle cells, for example, is very low (1 to 3 mm Hg) and nearly uniform. This pattern can be explained by the presence of myoglobin in the cell that acts as a reservoir for O_2 and enhances its diffusion within the cell.

How low can the tissue Po_2 fall before O_2 utilization ceases? In measurements on suspensions of liver mitochondria *in vitro*, O_2 consumption continues at the same rate until the Po_2 falls to the region of 3 mm Hg. Thus, it appears that the purpose of the much higher Po_2 in capillary blood is to

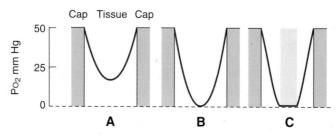

Figure 6-9. Scheme showing the fall of Po_2 between adjacent open capillaries. In *A*, oxygen delivery is adequate; in *B*, critical; and in *C*, inadequate for aerobic metabolism in the central core of tissue.

Table 6.1	Features of Different Types of Hypoxemia or Tissue Hypoxia[a]								
	PA_{O_2}	PA_{CO_2}	Pa_{O_2}	Pa_{CO_2}	Ca_{O_2}	Sa_{O_2}	$P\bar{v}_{O_2}$	$C\bar{v}_{O_2}$	O_2 Administration Helpful?
Lungs									
Hypoventilation	↓	↑	↓	↑	↓	↓	↓	↓	Yes
Diffusion impairment	O	O	↓	O	↓	↓	↓	↓	Yes
Shunt	O	O	↓	O	↓	↓	↓	↓	Yes[b]
$\dot{V}_A/\dot{Q}$ inequality	Varies	↑ or O	↓	↑ or O	↓	↓	↓	↓	Yes
Blood									
Anemia	O	O	O	O	↓	O	↓	↓	Yes[b]
CO poisoning	O	O	O	O	↓	O[c]	↓	↓	Yes[b]
Tissue									
Cyanide poisoning	O	O	O	O	O	O	↑	↑	No

[a]O, normal; ↑ increased; ↓ decreased.
[b]Of some (but limited) value because of increased dissolved oxygen.
[c]If O_2 saturation is calculated for hemoglobin not bound to CO.

ensure an adequate pressure for diffusion of O_2 to the mitochondria and that at the sites of O_2 utilization, the Po_2 may be very low.

An abnormally low Po_2 in tissues is called tissue hypoxia. This is frequently caused by low O_2 delivery, which can be expressed as the cardiac output multiplied by the arterial O_2 concentration, or $\dot{Q} \times Ca_{O_2}$. The factors that determine Ca_{O_2} were discussed on page 80. Tissue hypoxia can be due to (1) a low Po_2 in arterial blood caused, for example, by pulmonary disease ("hypoxic hypoxia"); (2) a reduced ability of blood to carry O_2, as in anemia or carbon monoxide poisoning ("anemic hypoxia"); or (3) a reduction in tissue blood flow, either generalized, as in shock, or because of local obstruction ("circulatory hypoxia"). A fourth cause is some toxic substance that interferes with the ability of the tissues to utilize available O_2 ("histotoxic hypoxia"). An example is cyanide, which prevents the use of O_2 by cytochrome oxidase. In this case, the O_2 concentration of venous blood is high and the O_2 consumption of the tissue extremely low, because these are related by the Fick principle as applied to peripheral O_2 consumption. Table 6-1 summarizes some of the features of the different types of hypoxemia and tissue hypoxia.

KEY CONCEPTS

1. Most of the O_2 transported in the blood is bound to hemoglobin. The maximum amount that can be bound is called the O_2 capacity. The O_2 saturation is the amount combined with hemoglobin divided by the capacity and is equal to the proportion of the binding sites that are occupied by O_2.
2. The O_2 dissociation curve is shifted to the right (that is, the O_2 affinity of the hemoglobin is reduced) by increases in Pco_2, H^+, temperature, and 2,3-diphosphoglycerate.

3. Most of the CO_2 in the blood is in the form of bicarbonate, with smaller amounts as dissolved and carbamino compounds.
4. The CO_2 dissociation curve is much steeper and more linear than that for O_2.
5. The acid-base status of the blood is determined by the Henderson-Hasselbalch equation and especially the ratio of bicarbonate concentration to the P_{CO_2}. Acid-base abnormalities include respiratory and metabolic acidosis and alkalosis.
6. The P_{O_2} in some tissues is less than 5 mm Hg, and the purpose of the much higher P_{O_2} in the capillary blood is to provide an adequate gradient for diffusion. Factors determining O_2 delivery to tissues include the blood O_2 concentration and the blood flow.

QUESTIONS

For each question, choose the one best answer.

1. The presence of hemoglobin in normal arterial blood increases its oxygen concentration approximately how many times?

   A. 10
   B. 30
   C. 50
   D. 70
   E. 90

2. An increase in which of the following increases the O_2 affinity of hemoglobin?

   A. Temperature
   B. P_{CO_2}
   C. H^+ concentration
   D. 2,3-DPG
   E. Carbon monoxide added to the blood

3. A patient with carbon monoxide poisoning is treated with hyperbaric oxygen that increases the arterial P_{O_2} to 2000 mm Hg. The amount of oxygen dissolved in the arterial blood (in $ml \cdot 100\ ml^{-1}$) is

   A. 2
   B. 3
   C. 4
   D. 5
   E. 6

4. A patient with severe anemia has normal lungs. You would expect

   A. Low arterial P_{O_2}.
   B. Low arterial O_2 saturation.
   C. Normal arterial O_2 concentration.
   D. Low oxygen concentration of mixed venous blood.
   E. Normal tissue P_{O_2}.

5. In carbon monoxide poisoning, you would expect

   A. Reduced arterial P_{O_2}.
   B. Normal oxygen concentration of arterial blood.
   C. Reduced oxygen concentration of mixed venous blood.
   D. O_2 dissociation curve is shifted to the right.
   E. Carbon monoxide has a distinct odor.

6. The laboratory reports the following arterial blood gas values in a patient with severe lung disease who is breathing air: Po_2 60 mm Hg, Pco_2 110 mm Hg, pH 7.20. You conclude

   A. The patient has a normal Po_2.
   B. The patient has a normal Pco_2.
   C. There is a respiratory alkalosis.
   D. There is a partially compensated respiratory alkalosis.
   E. The values for Po_2 and Pco_2 are internally inconsistent.

7. Most of the carbon dioxide transported in the arterial blood is in the form of

   A. Dissolved.
   B. Bicarbonate.
   C. Attached to hemoglobin.
   D. Carbamino compounds.
   E. Carbonic acid.

8. A patient with chronic lung disease has arterial Po_2 and Pco_2 values of 50 and 60 mm Hg, respectively, and a pH of 7.35. How is his acid-base status best described?

   A. Normal
   B. Partially compensated respiratory alkalosis
   C. Partially compensated respiratory acidosis
   D. Metabolic acidosis
   E. Metabolic alkalosis

9. The Po_2 (in mm Hg) inside skeletal muscle cells during exercise is closest to

   A. 3
   B. 10
   C. 20
   D. 30
   E. 40

10. A patient with chronic pulmonary disease undergoes emergency surgery. Postoperatively, the arterial Po_2, Pco_2, and pH are 50 mm Hg, 50 mm Hg, and 7.20, respectively. How would the acid-base status be best described?

    A. Mixed respiratory and metabolic acidosis
    B. Uncompensated respiratory acidosis
    C. Fully compensated respiratory acidosis
    D. Uncompensated metabolic acidosis
    E. Fully compensated metabolic acidosis

11. The laboratory provides the following report on arterial blood from a patient: Pco_2 32 mm Hg, pH 7.25, HCO_3 concentration 25 mmol·liter^{-1}. You conclude that there is

    A. Respiratory alkalosis with metabolic compensation.
    B. Acute respiratory acidosis.
    C. Metabolic acidosis with respiratory compensation.
    D. Metabolic alkalosis with respiratory compensation.
    E. A laboratory error.

12. A patient with shortness of breath is breathing air at sea level, and an arterial blood sample shows Po_2 90 mm Hg, Pco_2 32 mm Hg, pH 7.30. Assuming that the respiratory exchange ratio is 0.8, these data indicate

    A. Primary respiratory alkalosis with metabolic compensation.
    B. Normal alveolar-arterial Po_2 difference.
    C. Arterial O_2 saturation less than 70%.
    D. The sample was mistakenly taken from a vein.
    E. Partially compensated metabolic acidosis.

Mechanics of Breathing 7

▶ **HOW THE LUNG IS SUPPORTED AND MOVED**

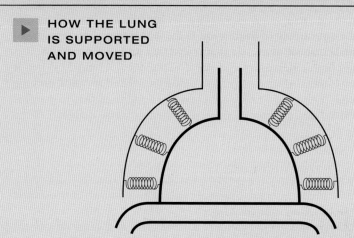

We saw in Chapter 2 that gas gets to and from the alveoli by the process of ventilation. We now turn to the forces that move the lung and chest wall, and the resistances that they overcome. First, we consider the muscles of respiration, both inspiration and expiration. Then we look at the factors determining the elastic properties of the lung, including the tissue elements and the air-liquid surface tension. Next, we examine the mechanism of regional differences in ventilation and also the closure of small airways. Just as the lung is elastic, so is the chest wall, and we look at the interaction between the two. The physical principles of airway resistance are then considered, along with its measurement, chief site in the lung, and physiological factors that affect it. Dynamic compression of the airways during a forced expiration is analyzed. Finally, the work required to move the lung and chest wall is considered.

▶ Muscles of Respiration

Inspiration

The most important muscle of inspiration is the *diaphragm*. This consists of a thin, dome-shaped sheet of muscle that is inserted into the lower ribs. It is supplied by the phrenic nerves from cervical segments 3, 4, and 5. When it contracts, the abdominal contents are forced downward and forward, and the vertical dimension of the chest cavity is increased. In addition, the rib margins are lifted and moved out, causing an increase in the transverse diameter of the thorax (Figure 7-1).

In normal tidal breathing, the level of the diaphragm moves about 1 cm or so, but on forced inspiration and expiration, a total excursion of up to 10 cm may occur. When the diaphragm is paralyzed, it moves *up* rather than *down* with inspiration because the intrathoracic pressure falls. This is known as *paradoxical movement* and can be demonstrated at fluoroscopy when the patient sniffs.

The *external intercostal muscles* connect adjacent ribs and slope downward and forward (Figure 7-2). When they contract, the ribs are pulled upward and forward, causing an increase in both the lateral and the anteroposterior diameters of the thorax. The lateral dimension increases because of the "bucket-handle" movement of the ribs. The intercostal muscles are supplied by intercostal nerves that come off the spinal cord at the same level. Paralysis of the intercostal muscles alone does not seriously affect breathing because the diaphragm is so effective.

The *accessory muscles of inspiration* include the scalene muscles, which elevate the first two ribs, and the sternomastoids, which raise the sternum. There is little, if any, activity in these muscles during quiet breathing, but during

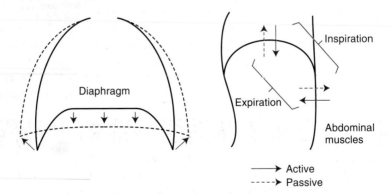

Figure 7-1. On inspiration, the dome-shaped diaphragm contracts, the abdominal contents are forced down and forward, and the rib cage is widened. Both increase the volume of the thorax. On forced expiration, the abdominal muscles contract and push the diaphragm up.

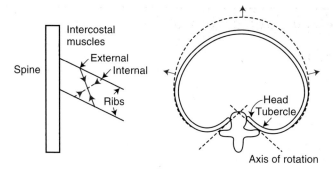

Figure 7-2. When the external intercostal muscles contract, the ribs are pulled upward and forward, and they rotate on an axis joining the tubercle and the head of a rib. As a result, both the lateral and anteroposterior diameters of the thorax increase. The internal intercostals have the opposite action.

exercise, they may contract vigorously. Other muscles that play a minor role include the alae nasi, which cause flaring of the nostrils, and small muscles in the neck and head.

Expiration

This is passive during quiet breathing. The lung and chest wall are elastic and tend to return to their equilibrium positions after being actively expanded during inspiration. During exercise and voluntary hyperventilation, expiration becomes active. The most important muscles of expiration are those of the *abdominal wall*, including the rectus abdominis, internal and external oblique muscles, and transversus abdominis. When these muscles contract, intra-abdominal pressure is raised, and the diaphragm is pushed upward. These muscles also contract forcefully during coughing, vomiting, and defecation.

The *internal intercostal muscles* assist active expiration by pulling the ribs downward and inward (opposite to the action of the external intercostal muscles), thus decreasing the thoracic volume. In addition, they stiffen the intercostal spaces to prevent them from bulging outward during straining. Experimental studies show that the actions of the respiratory muscles, especially the intercostals, are more complicated than this brief account suggests.

Respiratory Muscles

- Inspiration is active; expiration is passive during rest
- The diaphragm is the most important muscle of inspiration; it is supplied by phrenic nerves that originate high in the cervical region
- Other muscles include the intercostals, abdominal muscles, and accessory muscles

▶ Elastic Properties of the Lung

Pressure-Volume Curve

Suppose we take an excised animal lung, cannulate the trachea, and place it inside a jar (Figure 7-3). When the pressure within the jar is reduced below atmospheric pressure, the lung expands, and its change in volume can be measured with a spirometer. The pressure is held at each level, as indicated by the points, for a few seconds to allow the lung to come to rest. In this way, the pressure-volume curve of the lung can be plotted.

In Figure 7-3, the expanding pressure around the lung is generated by a pump, but in humans, it is developed by an increase in volume of the chest cage. The fact that the intrapleural space between the lung and the chest wall is much smaller than the space between the lung and the bottle in Figure 7-3 makes no essential difference. The intrapleural space contains only a few milliliters of fluid.

Figure 7-3 shows that the curves that the lung follows during inflation and deflation are different. This behavior is known as *hysteresis*. Note that the lung volume at any given pressure during deflation is larger than during inflation. Note also that the lung without any expanding pressure has some air inside it. In fact, even if the pressure around the lung is raised above atmospheric pressure, little further air is lost because small airways close, trapping gas in the alveoli (compare Figure 7-9). This *airway closure* occurs at higher lung volumes with increasing age and also in some types of lung disease.

In Figure 7-3, the pressure inside the airways and alveoli of the lung is the same as atmospheric pressure, which is zero on the horizontal axis. Thus, this

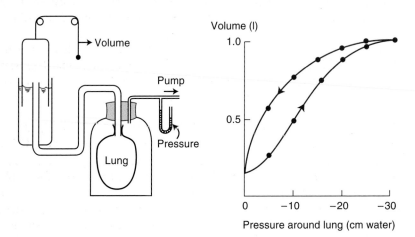

Figure 7-3. Measurement of the pressure-volume curve of excised lung. The lung is held at each pressure for a few seconds while its volume is measured. The curve is nonlinear and becomes flatter at high expanding pressures. Note that the inflation and deflation curves are not the same; this is called hysteresis.

axis also measures the difference in pressure between the inside and the outside of the lung. This is known as *transpulmonary pressure* and is numerically equal to the pressure around the lung when the alveolar pressure is atmospheric. It is also possible to measure the pressure-volume relationship of the lung shown in Figure 7-3 by inflating it with positive pressure and leaving the pleural surface exposed to the atmosphere. In this case, the horizontal axis could be labeled "airway pressure," and the values would be positive. The curves would be identical to those shown in Figure 7-3.

Compliance

The slope of the pressure-volume curve, or the volume change per unit pressure change, is known as the *compliance*. In the normal range (expanding pressure of about −5 to −10 cm water), the lung is remarkably distensible or very compliant. The compliance of the human lung is about 200 ml·cm water^{-1}. However, at high expanding pressures, the lung is stiffer, and its compliance is smaller, as shown by the flatter slope of the curve.

A *reduced* compliance is caused by an increase of fibrous tissue in the lung (pulmonary fibrosis). In addition, compliance is reduced by alveolar edema, which prevents the inflation of some alveoli. Compliance also falls if the lung remains unventilated for a long period, especially if its volume is low. This may be partly caused by atelectasis (collapse) of some units, but increases in surface tension also occur (see below). Compliance is also reduced somewhat if the pulmonary venous pressure is increased and the lung becomes engorged with blood.

An *increased* compliance occurs in pulmonary emphysema and in the normal aging lung. In both instances, an alteration in the elastic tissue in the lung is probably responsible. Increased compliance also occurs during an asthma attack, but the reason is unclear.

The compliance of a lung depends on its size. Clearly, the change in volume per unit change of pressure will be larger for a human lung than, say, a mouse lung. For this reason, the compliance per unit volume of lung, or *specific compliance*, is sometimes measured if we wish to draw conclusions about the intrinsic elastic properties of the lung tissue.

The pressure surrounding the lung is less than atmospheric in Figure 7-3 (and in the living chest) because of the elastic recoil of the lung. What is responsible for the lung's elastic behavior, that is, its tendency to return to its resting volume after distension? One factor is the elastic tissue, which is visible in histological sections. Fibers of elastin and collagen can be seen in the alveolar walls and around vessels and bronchi. Probably the elastic behavior of the lung has less to do with simple elongation of these fibers than it does with their geometrical arrangement. An analogy is a nylon stocking, which is very distensible because of its knitted makeup, although the individual nylon fibers are very difficult to stretch. The changes in elastic recoil that occur in the lung with age and in emphysema are presumably caused by changes in this elastic tissue.

Surface Tension

Another important factor in the pressure-volume behavior of lung is the surface tension of the liquid film lining the alveoli. Surface tension is the force (in dynes, for example) acting across an imaginary line 1 cm long in the surface of the liquid (Figure 7-4A). It arises because the attractive forces between adjacent molecules of the liquid are much stronger than those between the liquid and gas, with the result that the liquid surface area becomes as small as possible. This behavior is seen clearly in a soap bubble blown on the end of a tube (Figure 7-4B). The surfaces of the bubble contract as much as they can, forming a sphere (smallest surface area for a given volume) and generating a pressure that can be predicted from Laplace's law: pressure = (4 × surface tension)/radius. When only one surface is involved in a liquid-lined spherical alveolus, the numerator is 2 rather than 4.

Pressure-Volume Curve of the Lung

- Nonlinear, with the lung becoming stiffer at high volumes
- Shows hysteresis between inflation and deflation
- Compliance is the slope $\Delta V/\Delta P$
- Behavior depends on both structural proteins (collagen, elastin) and surface tension

---

The first evidence that surface tension might contribute to the pressure-volume behavior of the lung was obtained when it was found that lungs inflated with saline have a much larger compliance (are easier to distend) than air-filled lungs (Figure 7-5). Because the saline abolished the surface tension forces but presumably did not affect the tissue forces of the lung, this observation meant that surface tension contributed a large part of the static recoil force of the lung. Some time later, workers studying edema foam coming

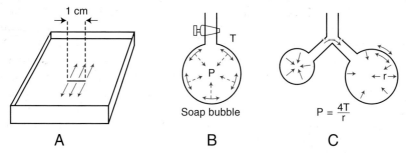

Soap bubble $P = \dfrac{4T}{r}$

A   B   C

Figure 7-4. **A.** Surface tension is the force (in dynes, for example) acting across an imaginary line 1 cm long in a liquid surface. **B.** Surface forces in a soap bubble tend to reduce the area of the surface and generate a pressure within the bubble. **C.** Because the smaller bubble generates a larger pressure, it blows up the larger bubble.

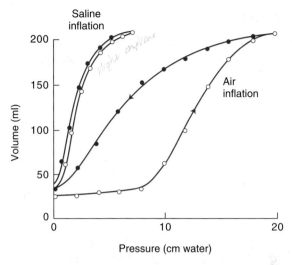

Figure 7-5. Comparison of pressure-volume curves of air-filled and saline-filled lungs (cat). *Open circles*, inflation; *closed circles*, deflation. Note that the saline-filled lung has a higher compliance and also much less hysteresis than the air-filled lung.

from the lungs of animals exposed to noxious gases noticed that the tiny air bubbles of the foam were extremely stable. They recognized that this indicated a very low surface tension, an observation that led to the remarkable discovery of pulmonary *surfactant*.

It is now known that some of the cells lining the alveoli secrete a material that profoundly lowers the surface tension of the alveolar lining fluid. Surfactant is a phospholipid, and dipalmitoyl phosphatidylcholine (DPPC) is an important constituent. Alveolar epithelial cells are of two types. Type I cells have the shape of a fried egg, with long cytoplasmic extensions spreading out thinly over the alveolar walls (Figure 1-1). Type II cells are more compact (Figure 7-6), and electron microscopy shows lamellated bodies within them that are extruded into the alveoli and transform into surfactant. Some of the surfactant can be washed out of animal lungs by rinsing them with saline.

The phospholipid DPPC is synthesized in the lung from fatty acids that are either extracted from the blood or are themselves synthesized in the lung. Synthesis is fast, and there is a rapid turnover of surfactant. If the blood flow to a region of lung is abolished as the result of an embolus, for example, the surfactant there may be depleted. Surfactant is formed relatively late in fetal life, and babies born without adequate amounts develop respiratory distress and may die.

The effects of this material on surface tension can be studied with a surface balance (Figure 7-7). This consists of a tray containing saline on which a small amount of test material is placed. The area of the surface is then alternately expanded and compressed by a movable barrier while the surface tension is

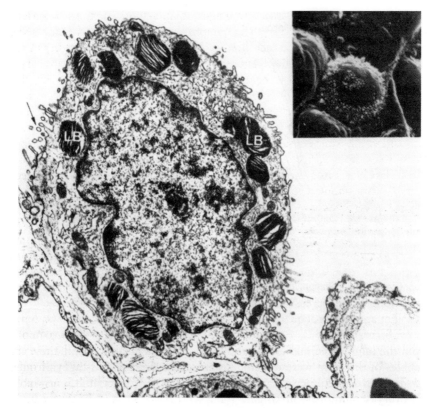

Figure 7-6. Electron micrograph of type II alveolar epithelial cell (×10,000). Note the lamellated bodies (LB), large nucleus, and microvilli (*arrows*). The *inset at top right* is a scanning electron micrograph showing the surface view of a type II cell with its characteristic distribution of microvilli (×3400).

measured from the force exerted on a platinum strip. Pure saline gives a surface tension of about 70 dynes·cm^{-1} (70 mN·m^{-1}), regardless of the area of its surface. Adding detergent reduces the surface tension, but again this is independent of area. When lung washings are placed on the saline, the curve shown in Figure 7-7B is obtained. Note that the surface tension changes greatly with the surface area and that there is hysteresis (compare Figure 7-3). Note also that the surface tension falls to extremely low values when the area is small.

How does surfactant reduce the surface tension so much? Apparently the molecules of DPPC are hydrophobic at one end and hydrophilic at the other, and they align themselves in the surface. When this occurs, their intermolecular repulsive forces oppose the normal attracting forces between the liquid surface molecules that are responsible for surface tension. The reduction in surface tension is greater when the film is compressed because the molecules of DPPC are then crowded closer together and repel each other more.

What are the physiological advantages of surfactant? First, a low surface tension in the alveoli increases the compliance of the lung and reduces the work of expanding it with each breath. Next, stability of the alveoli is promoted. The 500 million alveoli appear to be inherently unstable because areas of atelectasis (collapse) often form in the presence of disease. This is a complex subject, but one way of looking at the lung is to regard it as a collection of millions of tiny bubbles (although this is clearly an oversimplification). In such an arrangement, there is a tendency for small bubbles to collapse and blow up large ones. Figure 7-4C shows that the pressure generated by a given surface force in a bubble is inversely proportional to its radius, with the result that if the surface tensions are the same, the pressure inside a small bubble exceeds that in a large bubble. However, Figure 7-7 shows that when lung washings are present, a small surface area is associated with a small surface tension. Thus, the tendency for small alveoli to empty into large alveoli is apparently reduced.

A third role of surfactant is to help to keep the alveoli dry. Just as the surface tension forces tend to collapse alveoli, they also tend to suck fluid out of the capillaries. In effect, the surface tension of the curved alveolar surface reduces the hydrostatic pressure in the tissue outside the capillaries. By reducing these surface forces, surfactant prevents the transudation of fluid.

What are the consequences of loss of surfactant? On the basis of its functions discussed above, we would expect these to be stiff lungs (low compliance), areas of atelectasis, and alveoli filled with transudate. Indeed, these are the pathophysiological features of the infant respiratory distress syndrome, and this disease is caused by an absence of this crucial material. It is now possible to treat these newborns by instilling synthesized surfactant into the lung.

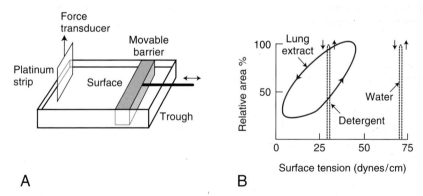

Figure 7-7. A. Surface balance. The area of the surface is altered, and the surface tension is measured from the force exerted on a platinum strip dipped into the surface. **B.** Plots of surface tension and area obtained with a surface balance. Note that lung washings show a change in surface tension with area and that the minimal tension is very small. The axes are chosen to allow a comparison with the pressure-volume curve of the lung (Figures 7-3 and 7-5).

There is another mechanism that apparently contributes to the stability of the alveoli in the lung. Figures 1-2, 1-7, and 4-3 remind us that all the alveoli (except those immediately adjacent to the pleural surface) are surrounded by other alveoli and are therefore supported by one another. In a structure such as this with many connecting links, any tendency for one group of units to reduce or increase its volume relative to the rest of the structure is opposed. For example, if a group of alveoli has a tendency to collapse, large expanding forces will be developed on them because the surrounding parenchyma is expanded.

Pulmonary Surfactant

- Reduces the surface tension of the alveolar lining layer
- Produced by type II alveolar epithelial cells
- Contains dipalmitoyl phosphatidylcholine
- Absence results in reduced lung compliance, alveolar atelectasis, and tendency to pulmonary edema

This support offered to lung units by those surrounding them is termed *interdependence*. The same factors explain the development of low pressures around large blood vessels and airways as the lung expands (Figure 4-2).

▶ Cause of Regional Differences in Ventilation

We saw in Figure 2-7 that the lower regions of the lung ventilate more than the upper zones, and this is a convenient place to discuss the cause of these topographical differences. It has been shown that the intrapleural pressure is less negative at the bottom than the top of the lung (Figure 7-8). The reason for this is the weight of the lung. Anything that is supported requires a larger pressure below it than above it to balance the downward-acting weight forces, and the lung, which is partly supported by the rib cage and diaphragm, is no exception. Thus, the pressure near the base is higher (less negative) than at the apex.

Figure 7-8 shows the way in which the volume of a portion of lung (e.g., a lobe) expands as the pressure around it is decreased (compare Figure 7-3). The pressure inside the lung is the same as atmospheric pressure. Note that the lung is easier to inflate at low volumes than at high volumes, where it becomes stiffer. Because the expanding pressure at the base of the lung is small, this region has a small resting volume. However, because it is situated on a steep part of the pressure-volume curve, it expands well on inspiration. By contrast, the apex of the lung has a large expanding pressure, a big resting volume, and small change in volume in inspiration.*

---

*This explanation is an oversimplification because the pressure-volume behavior of a portion of a structure such as the lung may not be identical to that of the whole organ.

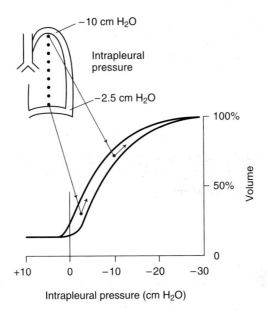

Figure 7-8. Explanation of the regional differences of ventilation down the lung. Because of the weight of the lung, the intrapleural pressure is less negative at the base than at the apex. As a consequence, the basal lung is relatively compressed in its resting state but expands more on inspiration than the apex.

Now when we talk of regional differences in ventilation, we mean the change in volume per unit resting volume. It is clear from Figure 7-8 that the base of the lung has both a larger change in volume and smaller resting volume than the apex. Thus, its ventilation is greater. Note the paradox that although the base of the lung is relatively poorly expanded compared with the apex, it is better ventilated. The same explanation can be given for the large ventilation of dependent lung in both the supine and lateral positions.

A remarkable change in the distribution of ventilation occurs at low lung volumes. Figure 7-9 is similar to Figure 7-8 except that it represents the situation at residual volume (RV) (i.e., after a full expiration; see Figure 2-2). Now the intrapleural pressures are less negative because the lung is not so well expanded and the elastic recoil forces are smaller. However, the differences between apex and base are still present because of the weight of the lung. Note that the intrapleural pressure at the base now actually exceeds airway (atmospheric) pressure. Under these conditions, the lung at the base is not being expanded but compressed, and ventilation is impossible until the local intrapleural pressure falls below atmospheric pressure. By contrast, the apex of the lung is on a favorable part of the pressure-volume curve and ventilates well. Thus, the normal distribution of ventilation is inverted, the upper regions ventilating better than the lower zones.

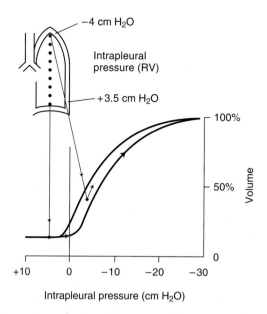

Figure 7-9. Situation at very low lung volumes. Now intrapleural pressures are less negative, and the pressure at the base actually exceeds airway (atmospheric) pressure. As a consequence, airway closure occurs in this region, and no gas enters with small inspirations.

Airway Closure

The compressed region of lung at the base does not have all its gas squeezed out. In practice, small airways, probably in the region of respiratory bronchioles (Figure 1-4), close first, thus trapping gas in the distal alveoli. This *airway closure* occurs only at very low lung volumes in young normal subjects. However, in elderly apparently normal people, airway closure in the lowermost regions of the lung occurs at higher volumes and may be present at functional residual capacity (FRC) (Figure 2-2). The reason is that the aging lung loses some of its elastic recoil, and intrapleural pressures therefore become less negative, thus approaching the situation shown in Figure 7-9. In these circumstances, dependent (that is, lowermost) regions of the lung may be only intermittently ventilated, and this leads to defective gas exchange (Chapter 5). A similar situation frequently develops in patients with some types of chronic lung disease.

▶ Elastic Properties of the Chest Wall

Just as the lung is elastic, so is the thoracic cage. This can be illustrated by putting air into the intrapleural space (pneumothorax). Figure 7-10 shows that the normal pressure outside the lung is subatmospheric just as it is in the jar of Figure 7-3. When air is introduced into the intrapleural space, raising the pressure to atmospheric, the lung collapses inward, and the chest wall springs outward. This shows that under equilibrium conditions, the chest wall is pulled inward while the lung is pulled outward, the two pulls balancing each other.

These interactions can be seen more clearly if we plot a pressure-volume curve for the lung and chest wall (Figure 7-11). For this, the subject inspires or expires from a spirometer and then relaxes the respiratory muscles while the airway pressure is measured ("relaxation pressure"). Incidentally, this is difficult for an untrained subject. Figure 7-11 shows that at FRC, the relaxation pressure of the lung plus chest wall is atmospheric. Indeed, FRC is the equilibrium volume when the elastic recoil of the lung is balanced by the normal tendency for the chest wall to spring out. At volumes above this, the pressure is positive, and at smaller volumes, the pressure is subatmospheric.

Figure 7-11 also shows the curve for the lung alone. This is similar to that shown in Figure 7-3, except that for clarity no hysteresis is indicated, and the pressures are positive instead of negative. They are the pressures that would be found from the experiment of Figure 7-3 if, after the lung had reached a certain volume, the line to the spirometer was clamped, the jar opened to the atmosphere (so that the lung relaxed against the closed airway), and the airway pressure measured. Note that at zero pressure the lung is at its *minimal volume*, which is below RV.

The third curve is for the chest wall only. We can imagine this being measured on a subject with a normal chest wall and no lung. Note that at FRC, the relaxation pressure is negative. In other words, at this volume the chest cage is tending to spring out. It is not until the volume is increased to about 75% of the vital capacity that the relaxation pressure is atmospheric, that is, that the chest wall has found its equilibrium position. At every volume, the relaxation pressure of the lung plus chest wall is the sum of the pressures for the lung and the chest wall measured separately. Because the pressure (at a given volume) is inversely proportional to compliance, this implies that the total compliance of the lung and chest wall is the sum of the reciprocals of the lung and chest wall compliances measured separately, or $1/C_T = 1/C_L + 1/C_{CW}$.

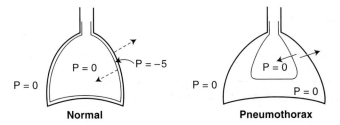

Figure 7-10. The tendency of the lung to recoil to its deflated volume is balanced by the tendency of the chest cage to bow out. As a result, the intrapleural pressure is subatmospheric. Pneumothorax allows the lung to collapse and the thorax to spring out.

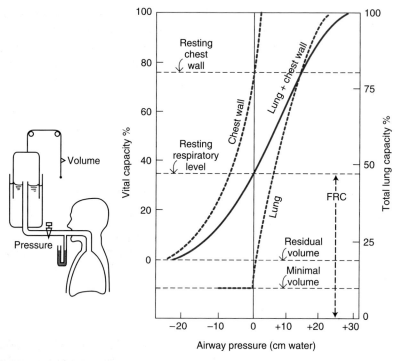

Figure 7-11. Relaxation pressure-volume curve of the lung and chest wall. The subject inspires (or expires) to a certain volume from the spirometer, the tap is closed, and the subject then relaxes his respiratory muscles. The curve for lung + chest wall can be explained by the addition of the individual lung and chest wall curves.

Relaxation Pressure-Volume Curve

- Elastic properties of both the lung and chest wall determine their combined volume
- At FRC, the inward pull of the lung is balanced by the outward spring of the chest wall
- Lung retracts at all volumes above minimal volume
- Chest wall tends to expand at volumes up to about 75% of vital capacity

---

▶ Airway Resistance

Airflow Through Tubes

If air flows through a tube (Figure 7-12), a difference of pressure exists between the ends. The pressure difference depends on the rate and pattern of flow. At low flow rates, the stream lines are parallel to the sides of the tube (A). This is known as laminar flow. As the flow rate is increased, unsteadiness develops, especially at branches. Here, separation of the stream lines from the wall may occur, with the formation of local eddies (B). At still higher flow rates, complete disorganization of the stream lines is seen; this is turbulence (C).

The pressure-flow characteristics for *laminar flow* were first described by the French physician Poiseuille. In straight circular tubes, the volume flow rate is given by

$$\dot{V} = \frac{P\pi r^4}{8nl}$$

where P is the driving pressure (ΔP in Figure 7-12A), r radius, n viscosity, and l length. It can be seen that driving pressure is proportional to flow rate, or $P = K\dot{V}$. Because flow resistance R is driving pressure divided by flow (compare p. 40), we have

$$R = \frac{8nl}{\pi r^4}$$

Note the critical importance of tube radius; if the radius is halved, the resistance increases 16-fold! However, doubling the length only doubles resistance. Note also that the viscosity of the gas, but not its density, affects the pressure-flow relationship under laminar flow conditions.

Another feature of laminar flow when it is fully developed is that the gas in the center of the tube moves twice as fast as the average velocity. Thus, a spike

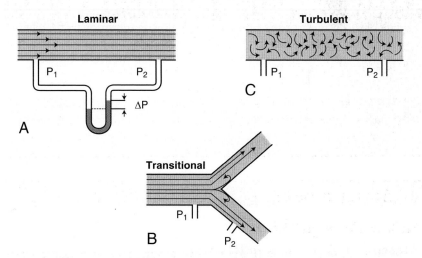

Figure 7-12. Patterns of airflow in tubes. In **A,** the flow is laminar; in **B,** transitional with eddy formation at branches; and in **C,** turbulent. Resistance is ($P_1 - P_2$)/flow.

of rapidly moving gas travels down the axis of the tube (Figure 7-12A). This changing velocity across the diameter of the tube is known as the *velocity profile*.

Turbulent flow has different properties. Here pressure is not proportional to flow rate but, approximately, to its square: $P = K\dot{V}^2$. In addition, the viscosity of the gas becomes relatively unimportant, but an increase in gas density increases the pressure drop for a given flow. Turbulent flow does not have the high axial flow velocity that is characteristic of laminar flow.

Whether flow will be laminar or turbulent depends to a large extent on the Reynolds number, Re. This is given by

$$Re = \frac{2rvd}{n}$$

where d is density, v average velocity, r radius, and n viscosity. Because density and velocity are in the numerator, and viscosity is in the denominator, the expression gives the ratio of inertial to viscous forces. In straight, smooth tubes, turbulence is probable when the Reynolds number exceeds 2000. The expression shows that turbulence is most likely to occur when the velocity of flow is high and the tube diameter is large (for a given velocity). Note also that a low-density gas such as helium tends to produce less turbulence.

In such a complicated system of tubes as the bronchial tree with its many branches, changes in caliber, and irregular wall surfaces, the application of the above principles is difficult. In practice, for laminar flow to occur, the entrance conditions of the tube are critical. If eddy formation occurs upstream at a branch point, this disturbance is carried downstream some distance before it disappears. Thus, in a rapidly branching system such as the lung, fully developed laminar flow (Figure 7-12A) probably only occurs in the very small airways where the Reynolds numbers are very low (~1 in terminal bronchioles). In most of the bronchial tree, flow is transitional (*B*), whereas true turbulence may occur in the trachea, especially on exercise when flow velocities are high. In general, driving pressure is determined by both the flow rate and its square: $P = K_1\dot{V} + K_2\dot{V}^2$.

Laminar and Turbulent Flow

- In laminar flow, resistance is inversely proportional to the fourth power of the radius of the tube
- In laminar flow, the velocity profile shows a central spike of fast gas
- Turbulent flow is most likely to occur at high Reynolds numbers, that is, when inertial forces dominate over viscous forces

Measurement of Airway Resistance

Airway resistance is the pressure difference between the alveoli and the mouth divided by a flow rate (Figure 7-12). Mouth pressure is easily measured with a manometer. Alveolar pressure can be deduced from measurements made in a body plethysmograph. More information on this technique is given on p. 169.

Pressures During the Breathing Cycle

Suppose we measure the pressures in the intrapleural and alveolar spaces during normal breathing.[†] Figure 7-13 shows that before inspiration begins, the intrapleural pressure is –5 cm water because of the elastic recoil of the lung (compare Figures 7-3 and 7-10). Alveolar pressure is zero (atmospheric) because with no airflow, there is no pressure drop along the airways. However, for inspiratory flow to occur, the alveolar pressure falls, thus establishing the driving pressure (Figure 7-12). Indeed, the extent of the fall depends on the flow rate and the resistance of the airways. In normal subjects, the change in alveolar pressure is only 1 cm water or so, but in patients with airway obstruction, it may be many times that.

Intrapleural pressure falls during inspiration for two reasons. First, as the lung expands, its elastic recoil increases (Figure 7-3). This alone would cause the intrapleural pressure to move along the broken line ABC. In addition, however, the reduction in alveolar pressure causes a further fall in intrapleural pressure,[‡] represented by the hatched area, so that the actual path is AB'C. Thus, the vertical distance between lines ABC and AB'C reflects the alveolar pressure at any instant. As an equation of pressures, (mouth – intrapleural) = (mouth – alveolar) + (alveolar – intrapleural).

On expiration, similar changes occur. Now intrapleural pressure is *less* negative than it would be in the absence of airway resistance because alveolar pressure is positive. Indeed, with a forced expiration, intrapleural pressure goes above zero.

Note that the shape of the alveolar pressure tracing is similar to that of flow. Indeed, they would be identical if the airway resistance remained constant during the cycle. Also, the intrapleural pressure curve ABC would have the same shape as the volume tracing if the lung compliance remained constant.

Chief Site of Airway Resistance

As the airways penetrate toward the periphery of the lung, they become more numerous but much narrower (see Figures 1-3 and 1-5). Based on Poiseuille's equation with its (radius)^4 term, it would be natural to think that the major part of the resistance lies in the very narrow airways. Indeed, this was thought to be the case for many years. However, it has now been shown by direct measurements of the pressure drop along the bronchial tree that the major site of resistance is the medium-sized bronchi and that the very small bronchioles contribute relatively little resistance. Figure 7-14 shows that most of

---

[†]Intrapleural pressure can be estimated by placing a balloon catheter in the esophagus.
[‡]There is also a contribution made by tissue resistance, which is considered later in this chapter.

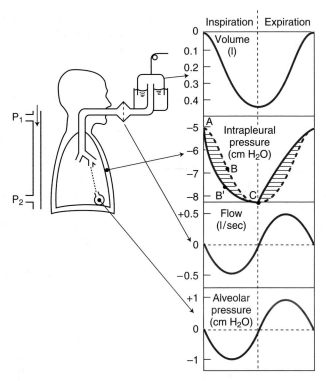

Figure 7-13. Pressures during the breathing cycle. If there was no airway resistance, alveolar pressure would remain at zero, and intrapleural pressure would follow the *broken line* ABC, which is determined by the elastic recoil of the lung. The fall in alveolar pressure is responsible for the *hatched* portion of intrapleural pressure (see text).

the pressure drop occurs in the airways up to the seventh generation. Less than 20% can be attributed to airways less than 2 mm in diameter (about generation 8). The reason for this apparent paradox is the prodigious number of small airways.

The fact that the peripheral airways contribute so little resistance is important in the detection of early airway disease. Because they constitute a "silent zone," it is probable that considerable small airway disease can be present before the usual measurements of airway resistance can detect an abnormality. This issue is considered in more detail in Chapter 10.

Factors Determining Airway Resistance

Lung volume has an important effect on airway resistance. Like the extra-alveolar blood vessels (Figure 4-2), the bronchi are supported by the radial traction of the surrounding lung tissue, and their caliber is increased as the lung expands (compare Figure 4-6). Figure 7-15 shows that as lung volume is reduced, airway resistance rises rapidly. If the reciprocal of resistance (conductance) is plotted against lung volume, an approximately linear relationship is obtained.

At very low lung volumes, the small airways may close completely, especially at the bottom of the lung, where the lung is less well expanded (Figure 7-9). Patients who have increased airway resistance often breathe at high lung volumes; this helps to reduce their airway resistance.

Contraction of *bronchial smooth muscle* narrows the airways and increases airway resistance. This may occur reflexly through the stimulation of receptors in the trachea and large bronchi by irritants such as cigarette smoke. Motor innervation is by the vagus nerve. The tone of the smooth muscle is under the control of the autonomic nervous system. Stimulation of adrenergic receptors causes bronchodilatation, as do epinephrine and isoproterenol.

β-Adrenergic receptors are of two types: β_1 receptors occur principally in the heart, whereas β_2 receptors relax smooth muscle in the bronchi, blood vessels, and uterus. Selective β_2-adrenergic agonists are now extensively used in the treatments of asthma.

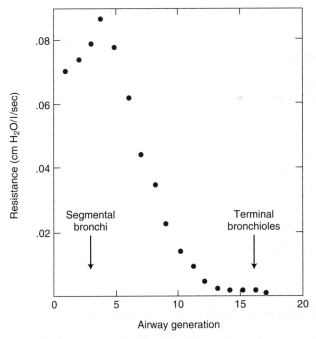

Figure 7-14. Location of the chief site of airway resistance. Note that the intermediate-sized bronchi contribute most of the resistance and that relatively little is located in the very small airways.

Parasympathetic activity causes bronchoconstriction, as does acetylcholine. A fall of P_{CO_2} in alveolar gas causes an increase in airway resistance, apparently as a result of a direct action on bronchiolar smooth muscle. The injection of histamine into the pulmonary artery causes constriction of smooth muscle located in the alveolar ducts.

The *density and viscosity* of the inspired gas affect the resistance offered to flow. The resistance is increased during a deep dive because the increased pressure raises gas density, but the increase is less when a helium-O_2 mixture is breathed. The fact that changes in density rather than viscosity have such an influence on resistance is evidence that flow is not purely laminar in the medium-sized airways, where the main site of resistance lies (Figure 7-14).

Airway Resistance

- Highest in the medium-sized bronchi; low in the very small airways
- Decreases as lung volume rises because the airways are then pulled open
- Bronchial smooth muscle is controlled by the autonomic nervous system; stimulation of β-adrenergic receptors causes bronchodilatation
- Breathing a dense gas, as when diving, increases resistance

Dynamic Compression of Airways

Suppose a subject inspires to total lung capacity and then exhales as hard as possible to RV. We can record a *flow-volume curve* like A in Figure 7-16, which

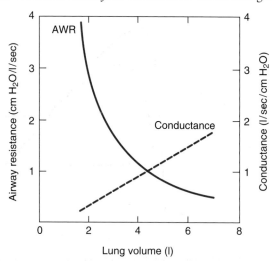

Figure 7-15. Variation of airway resistance (AWR) with lung volume. If the reciprocal of airway resistance (conductance) is plotted, the graph is a straight line.

shows that flow rises very rapidly to a high value but then declines over most of expiration. A remarkable feature of this flow-volume envelope is that it is virtually impossible to penetrate it. For example, no matter whether we start exhaling slowly and then accelerate, as in B, or make a less forceful expiration, as in C, the descending portion of the flow-volume curve takes virtually the same path. Thus, something powerful is limiting expiratory flow, and over most of the lung volume, flow rate is independent of effort.

We can get more information about this curious state of affairs by plotting the data in another way, as shown in Figure 7-17. For this, the subject takes a *series* of maximal inspirations (or expirations) and then exhales (or inhales) fully with varying degrees of effort. If the flow rates and intrapleural pressures are plotted at the *same* lung volume for each expiration and inspiration, so-called *isovolume pressure-flow curves* can be obtained. It can be seen that at high lung volumes, the expiratory flow rate continues to increase with effort, as might be expected. However, at mid or low volumes, the flow rate reaches a plateau and cannot be increased with further increase in intrapleural pressure. Under these conditions, flow is therefore *effort independent.*

The reason for this remarkable behavior is compression of the airways by intrathoracic pressure. Figure 7-18 shows schematically the forces acting across an airway within the lung. The pressure outside the airway is shown as intrapleural, although this is an oversimplification. In A, before inspiration has begun, airway pressure is everywhere zero (no flow), and because intrapleural pressure is –5 cm water, there is a pressure of 5 cm water holding the airway open. As inspiration starts (B), both intrapleural and alveolar pressure fall by 2 cm water (same lung volume as *A*, and tissue resistance is neglected), and flow begins. Because of the pressure drop along the airway, the pressure

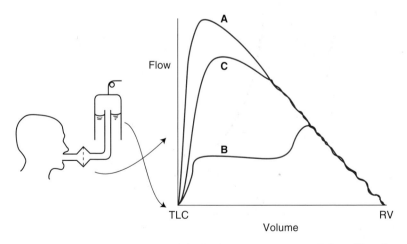

Figure 7-16. Flow-volume curves. In A, a maximal inspiration was followed by a forced expiration. In B, expiration was initially slow and then forced. In C, expiratory effort was submaximal. In all three, the descending portions of the curves are almost superimposed.

inside is –1 cm water, and there is a pressure of 6 cm water holding the airway open. At end-inspiration (C), again flow is zero, and there is an airway transmural pressure of 8 cm water.

Finally, at the onset of forced expiration (D), both intrapleural pressure and alveolar pressure increase by 38 cm water (same lung volume as C). Because of the pressure drop along the airway as flow begins, there is now a pressure of 11 cm water, tending to *close* the airway. Airway compression occurs, and the downstream pressure limiting flow becomes the pressure outside the airway, or intrapleural pressure. Thus, the effective driving pressure becomes alveolar minus intrapleural pressure. This is the same Starling resistor mechanism that limits the blood flow in zone 2 of the lung, where venous pressure becomes unimportant just as mouth pressure does here (Figures 4-8 and 4-9). Note that if intrapleural pressure is raised further by increased muscular effort in an attempt to expel gas, the effective driving pressure is unaltered because the difference between alveolar and intrapleural pressure is determined by lung volume. Thus, flow is independent of effort.

Maximal flow decreases with lung volume (Figure 7-16) because the difference between alveolar and intrapleural pressure decreases and the

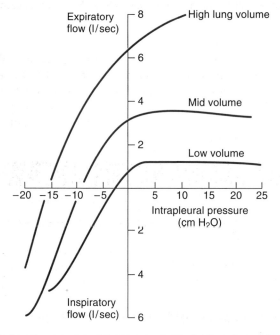

Figure 7-17. Isovolume pressure-flow curves drawn for three lung volumes. Each of these was obtained from a series of forced expirations and inspirations (see text). Note that at the high lung volume, a rise in intrapleural pressure (obtained by increasing expiratory effort) results in a greater expiratory flow. However, at mid and low volumes, flow becomes independent of effort after a certain intrapleural pressure has been exceeded.

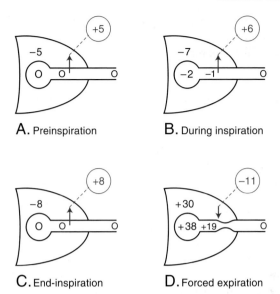

Figure 7-18. Scheme showing why airways are compressed during forced expiration. Note that the pressure difference across the airway is holding it open, except during a forced expiration. See text for details.

airways become narrower. Note also that flow is independent of the resistance of the airways downstream of the point of collapse, called the *equal pressure point*. As expiration progresses, the equal pressure point moves distally, deeper into the lung. This occurs because the resistance of the airways rises as lung volume falls, and therefore, the pressure within the airways falls more rapidly with distance from the alveoli.

Dynamic Compression of Airways

- Limits air flow in normal subjects during a forced expiration
- May occur in diseased lungs at relatively low expiratory flow rates, thus reducing exercise ability
- During dynamic compression, flow is determined by alveolar pressure minus pleural pressure (not mouth pressure) and is therefore independent of effort
- Is exaggerated in some lung diseases by reduced lung elastic recoil and loss of radial traction on airways

Several factors exaggerate this flow-limiting mechanism. One is any increase in resistance of the peripheral airways because that magnifies the pressure drop along them and thus decreases the intrabronchial pressure during expiration (19 cm water in D). Another is a low lung volume because that reduces the driving pressure (alveolar-intrapleural). This driving pressure is also reduced if recoil pressure is reduced, as in emphysema. Also in this disease, radial traction on the airways is reduced and they are compressed more readily. Indeed, while this type of flow limitation is seen only during forced expiration in normal subjects, it may occur during the expirations of normal breathing in patients with severe lung disease.

In the pulmonary function laboratory, information about airway resistance in a patient with lung disease can be obtained by measuring the flow rate during a maximal expiration. Figure 7-19 shows the spirometer record obtained when a subject inspires maximally and then exhales as hard and as completely as he or she can. The volume exhaled in the first second is called the forced expiratory volume, or $FEV_{1.0}$, and the total volume exhaled is the forced vital capacity, or FVC (this is often slightly less than the vital capacity measured on a slow exhalation as in Figure 2-2). Normally, the $FEV_{1.0}$ is about 80% of the FVC.

In disease, two general patterns can be distinguished. In *restrictive* diseases such as pulmonary fibrosis, both FEV and FVC are reduced, but characteristically the $FEV_{1.0}$/FVC% is normal or increased. In *obstructive* diseases such as chronic obstructive pulmonary disease or bronchial asthma, the $FEV_{1.0}$ is reduced much more than the FVC, giving a low FEV/FVC%. Frequently, mixed restrictive and obstructive patterns are seen.

A related measurement is the *forced expiratory flow rate*, or $FEF_{25-75\%}$, which is the average flow rate measured over the middle half of the expiration. Generally, this is closely related to the $FEV_{1.0}$, although occasionally it is reduced when the $FEV_{1.0}$ is normal. Sometimes other indices are also measured from the forced expiration curve.

Forced Expiration Test

- Measures the FEV and the FVC
- Simple to do and often informative
- Distinguishes between obstructive and restrictive disease

▶ Causes of Uneven Ventilation

The cause of the regional differences in ventilation in the lung was discussed on p. 105. Apart from these topographical differences, there is some additional inequality of ventilation at any given vertical level in the normal lung, and this is exaggerated in many diseases.

One mechanism of uneven ventilation is shown in Figure 7-20. If we regard a lung unit (Figure 2-1) as an elastic chamber connected to the atmosphere by a tube, the amount of ventilation depends on the compliance of the

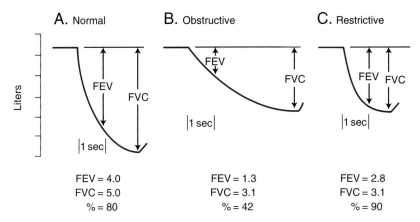

Figure 7-19. Measurement of forced expiratory volume ($FEB_{1.0}$) and forced vital capacity (FVC).

chamber and the resistance of the tube. In Figure 7-20, unit *A* has a normal distensibility and airway resistance. It can be seen that its volume change on inspiration is large and rapid so that it is complete before expiration for the whole lung begins (*broken line*). By contrast, unit *B* has a low compliance, and its change in volume is rapid but small. Finally, unit *C* has a large airway resistance so that inspiration is slow and not complete before the lung has begun to exhale. Note that the shorter the time available for inspiration (fast breathing rate), the smaller the inspired volume. Such a unit is said to have a long *time constant*, the value of which is given by the product of the compliance and resistance. Thus, inequality of ventilation can result from alterations in either local distensibility or airway resistance, and the pattern of inequality will depend on the frequency of breathing.

Another possible mechanism of uneven ventilation is incomplete diffusion within the airways of the respiratory zone (Figure 1-4). We saw in Chapter 1 that the dominant mechanism of ventilation of the lung beyond the terminal bronchioles is diffusion. Normally, this occurs so rapidly that differences in gas concentration in the acinus are virtually abolished within a fraction of a second. However, if there is dilation of the airways in the region of the respiratory bronchioles, as in some diseases, the distance to be covered by diffusion may be enormously increased. In these circumstances, inspired gas is not distributed uniformly within the respiratory zone because of uneven ventilation *along* the lung units.

▶ Tissue Resistance

When the lung and chest wall are moved, some pressure is required to overcome the viscous forces within the tissues as they slide over each other. Thus,

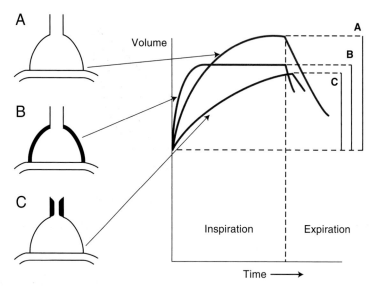

Figure 7-20. Effects of decreased compliance **(B)** and increased airway resistance **(C)** on ventilation of lung units compared with normal **(A)**. In both instances, the inspired volume is abnormally low.

part of the hatched portion of Figure 7-13 should be attributed to these tissue forces. However, this tissue resistance is only about 20% of the total (tissue + airway) resistance in young normal subjects, although it may increase in some diseases. This total resistance is sometimes called *pulmonary resistance* to distinguish it from airway resistance.

▶ Work of Breathing

Work is required to move the lung and chest wall. In this context, it is most convenient to measure work as pressure × volume.

Work Done on the Lung

This can be illustrated on a pressure-volume curve (Figure 7-21). During inspiration, the intrapleural pressure follows the curve ABC, and the work done on the lung is given by the area 0ABCD0. Of this, the trapezoid 0AECD0 represents the work required to overcome the elastic forces, and the hatched area ABCEA represents the work overcoming viscous (airway and tissue) resistance (compare Figure 7-13). The higher the airway resistance or the inspiratory flow rate, the more negative (rightward) would be the intrapleural pressure excursion between *A* and *C* and the larger the area.

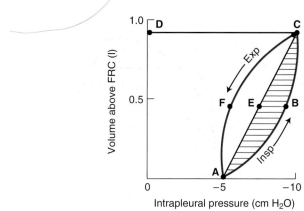

Figure 7-21. Pressure-volume curve of the lung showing the inspiratory work done overcoming elastic forces (*area 0AECD0*) and viscous forces (*hatched area ABCEA*).

On expiration, the area AECFA is work required to overcome airway (+ tissue) resistance. Normally, this falls within the trapezoid 0AECD0, and thus this work can be accomplished by the energy stored in the expanded elastic structures and released during a passive expiration. The difference between the areas AECFA and 0AECD0 represents the work dissipated as heat.

The higher the breathing rate, the faster the flow rates and the larger the viscous work area ABCEA. On the other hand, the larger the tidal volume, the larger the elastic work area 0AECD0. It is of interest that patients who have a reduced compliance (stiff lungs) tend to take small rapid breaths, whereas patients with severe airway obstruction sometimes breathe slowly. These patterns tend to reduce the work done on the lungs.

Total Work of Breathing

The total work done moving the lung and chest wall is difficult to measure, although estimates have been obtained by artificially ventilating paralyzed patients (or "completely relaxed" volunteers) in an iron-lung type of ventilator. Alternatively, the total work can be calculated by measuring the O_2 cost of breathing and assuming a figure for the efficiency as given by

$$\text{Efficiency \%} = \frac{\text{Useful work}}{\text{Total energy expended (or } O_2 \text{ cost)}} \times 100$$

The efficiency is believed to be about 5% to 10%.

The O_2 cost of quiet breathing is extremely small, being less than 5% of the total resting O_2 consumption. With voluntary hyperventilation, it is possible to increase this to 30%. In patients with obstructive lung disease, the O_2 cost of breathing may limit their exercise ability.

KEY CONCEPTS

1. Inspiration is active, but expiration during rest is passive. The most important muscle of respiration is the diaphragm.
2. The pressure-volume curve of the lung is nonlinear and shows hysteresis. The recoil pressure of the lung is attributable to both its elastic tissue and the surface tension of the alveolar lining layer.
3. Pulmonary surfactant is a phospholipid produced by type II alveolar epithelial cells. If the surfactant system is immature, as in some premature babies, the lung has a low compliance and is unstable and edematous.
4. The chest wall is elastic like the lung but normally tends to expand. At FRC, the inward recoil of the lung and the outward recoil of the chest wall are balanced.
5. In laminar flow as exists in small airways, the resistance is inversely proportional to the fourth power of the radius.
6. Lung airway resistance is reduced by increasing lung volume. If airway smooth muscle is contracted, as in asthma, the resistance is reduced by β_2-adrenergic agonists.
7. Dynamic compression of the airways during a forced expiration results in flow that is effort-independent. The driving pressure is then alveolar minus intrapleural pressure. In patients with chronic obstructive lung disease, dynamic compression can occur during mild exercise, thus causing severe disability.

QUESTIONS

For each question, choose the one best answer.

1. Concerning contraction of the diaphragm,

    A. The nerves that are responsible emerge from the spinal cord at the level of the lower thorax.
    B. It tends to flatten the diaphragm.
    C. It reduces the lateral distance between the lower rib margins.
    D. It causes the anterior abdominal wall to move in.
    E. It raises intrapleural pressure.

2. Concerning the pressure-volume behavior of the lung,

    A. Compliance decreases with age.
    B. Filling an animal lung with saline decreases compliance.
    C. Removing a lobe reduces total pulmonary compliance.
    D. Absence of surfactant increases compliance.
    E. In the upright lung at FRC, for a given change in intrapleural pressure, the alveoli near the base of the lung expand less than those near the apex.

3. Two bubbles have the same surface tension, but bubble X has 3 times the diameter of bubble Y. The ratio of the pressure in bubble X to that in bubble Y is

    A. 0.3:1
    B. 0.9:1
    C. 1:1
    D. 3:1
    E. 9:1

4. Pulmonary surfactant is produced by

A. Alveolar macrophages.
B. Goblet cells.
C. Leukocytes.
D. Type I alveolar cells.
E. Type II alveolar cells.

5. The basal regions of the upright human lung are normally better ventilated than the upper regions because

A. Airway resistance of the upper regions is higher than of the lower regions.
B. There is less surfactant in the upper regions.
C. The blood flow to the lower regions is higher.
D. The lower regions have a small resting volume and a relatively large increase in volume.
E. The P_{CO_2} of the lower regions is relatively high.

6. Pulmonary surfactant

A. Increases the surface tension of the alveolar lining liquid.
B. Is secreted by type I alveolar epithelial cells.
C. Is a protein.
D. Increases the work required to expand the lung.
E. Helps to prevent transudation of fluid from the capillaries into the alveolar spaces.

7. Concerning normal expiration during resting conditions,

A. Expiration is generated by the expiratory muscles.
B. Alveolar pressure is less than atmospheric pressure.
C. Intrapleural pressure gradually falls (becomes more negative) during the expiration.
D. Flow velocity of the gas (in cm·s⁻¹) in the large airways exceeds that in the terminal bronchioles.
E. Diaphragm moves down as expiration proceeds.

8. An anesthetized patient with paralyzed respiratory muscles and normal lungs is ventilated by positive pressure. If the anesthesiologist increases the lung volume 2 liters above FRC and holds the lung at that volume for 5 seconds, the most likely combination of pressures (in cm H_2O) is likely to be

	Mouth	Alveolar	Intrapleural
A.	0	0	−5
B.	0	+10	−5
C.	+10	+10	−10
D.	+20	+20	+5
E.	+10	0	−10

9. When a normal subject develops a spontaneous pneumothorax of his right lung, you would expect the following to occur:

A. Right lung contracts.
B. Chest wall on the right contracts.
C. Diaphragm on the right moves up.
D. Mediastinum moves to the right.
E. Blood flow to the right lung increases.

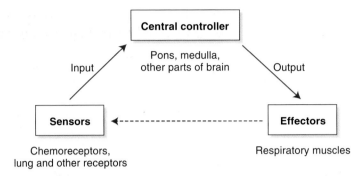

Figure 8-1. Basic elements of the respiratory control system. Information from various sensors is fed to the central controller, the output of which goes to the respiratory muscles. By changing ventilation, the respiratory muscles reduce perturbations of the sensors (negative feedback).

The three basic elements of the respiratory control system (Figure 8-1) are

1. *Sensors* that gather information and feed it to the

2. *Central controller* in the brain, which coordinates the information and, in turn, sends impulses to the

3. *Effectors* (respiratory muscles), which cause ventilation.

We shall see that increased activity of the effectors generally ultimately decreases the sensory input to the brain, for example, by decreasing the arterial P_{CO_2}. This is an example of negative feedback.

▶ Central Controller

The normal automatic process of breathing originates in impulses that come from the brainstem. The cortex can override these centers if voluntary control is desired. Additional input from other parts of the brain occurs under certain conditions.

Brainstem

The periodic nature of inspiration and expiration is controlled by the central pattern generator that comprises groups of neurons located in the pons and medulla. Three main groups of neurons are recognized.

1. *Medullary respiratory center* in the reticular formation of the medulla beneath the floor of the fourth ventricle. There is a group of cells in the ventrolateral region known as the *Pre-Botzinger Complex* that appears to be essential for the generation of the respiratory rhythm. In addition, a group of cells in the dorsal region of the medulla (*Dorsal Respiratory Group*) is chiefly associated with inspiration, and another group (*Ventral Respiratory Group*) is associated with expiration. These groups of cells have the property of intrinsic periodic firing and are responsible for the basic rhythm of ventilations. When all known afferent stimuli have been abolished, these cells generate repetitive bursts of action potentials that result in nervous impulses going to the diaphragm and other inspiratory muscles.

The intrinsic rhythm pattern of the inspiratory area starts with a latent period of several seconds during which there is no activity. Action potentials then begin to appear, increasing in a crescendo over the next few seconds. During this time, inspiratory muscle activity becomes stronger in a "ramp"-type pattern. Finally, the inspiratory action potentials cease, and inspiratory muscle tone falls to its preinspiratory level.

The inspiratory ramp can be "turned off" prematurely by inhibiting impulses from the *pneumotaxic center* (see below). In this way, inspiration is shortened and, as a consequence, the breathing rate increases. The output of the inspiratory cells is further modulated by impulses from the vagal and glossopharyngeal nerves. Indeed, these terminate in the tractus solitarius, which is situated close to the inspiratory area.

The *expiratory area* is quiescent during normal quiet breathing because ventilation is then achieved by active contraction of inspiratory muscles (chiefly the diaphragm), followed by passive relaxation of the chest wall to its equilibrium position (Chapter 7). However, in more forceful breathing, for example, on exercise, expiration becomes active as a result of the activity of the expiratory cells. Note that there is still not universal agreement on how the intrinsic rhythmicity of respiration is brought about by the medullary centers.

2. *Apneustic center* in the lower pons. This area is so named because if the brain of an experimental animal is sectioned just above this site, prolonged inspiratory gasps (apneuses) interrupted by transient expiratory efforts are seen. Apparently, the impulses from the center have an excitatory effect on the inspiratory area of the medulla, tending to prolong the ramp action potentials. Whether this apneustic center plays a role in normal human respiration is not known, although in some types of severe brain injury, this type of abnormal breathing is seen.

3. *Pneumotaxic center* in the upper pons. As indicated above, this area appears to "switch off" or inhibit inspiration and thus regulate inspiration volume and, secondarily, respiratory rate. This has been demonstrated experimentally in animals by direct electrical stimulation of the pneumotaxic center. Some investigators believe that the role of this center is "fine tuning" of respiratory rhythm because a normal rhythm can exist in the absence of this center.

Respiratory Centers

- Responsible for generating the rhythmic pattern of inspiration and expiration
- Located in the medulla and pons of the brainstem
- Receive input from chemoreceptors, lung and other receptors, and the cortex
- Major output is to the phrenic nerves, but there are also impulses to other respiratory muscles

Cortex

Breathing is under voluntary control to a considerable extent, and the cortex can override the function of the brainstem within limits. It is not difficult to halve the arterial P_{CO_2} by hyperventilation, although the consequent alkalosis may cause tetany with contraction of the muscles of the hand and foot (carpopedal spasm). Halving the P_{CO_2} in this way increases the arterial pH by about 0.2 unit (Figure 6-8).

Voluntary hypoventilation is more difficult. The duration of breath-holding is limited by several factors, including the arterial P_{CO_2} and P_{O_2}. A preliminary period of hyperventilation increases breath-holding time, especially if oxygen is breathed. However, factors other than chemical are involved. This is shown by the observation that if, at the breaking point of breath-holding, a gas mixture is inhaled that *raises* the arterial P_{CO_2} and *lowers* the P_{O_2}, a further period of breath-holding is possible.

Other Parts of the Brain

Other parts of the brain, such as the limbic system and hypothalamus, can alter the pattern of breathing, for example, in emotional states such as rage and fear.

▶ Effectors

The muscles of respiration include the diaphragm, intercostal muscles, abdominal muscles, and accessory muscles such as the sternomastoids. The actions of these were described at the beginning of Chapter 7. In the context of the control of ventilation, it is crucially important that these various muscle groups work in a coordinated manner; this is the responsibility of the central controller. There is evidence that some newborn children, particularly those who are premature, have uncoordinated respiratory muscle activity, especially during sleep. For example, the thoracic muscles may try to inspire while the abdominal muscles expire. This may be a factor in sudden infant death syndrome.

▶ Sensors

Central Chemoreceptors

A chemoreceptor is a receptor that responds to a change in the chemical composition of the blood or other fluid around it. The most important receptors involved in the minute-by-minute control of ventilation are those situated near the ventral surface of the medulla in the vicinity of the exit of the 9th and 10th nerves. In animals, local application of H^+ or dissolved CO_2 to this area stimulates breathing within a few seconds. At one time, it was thought that the medullary respiratory center itself was the site of action of CO_2, but it is now accepted that the chemoreceptors are anatomically separate. Some evidence suggests that they lie about 200 to 400 mm below the ventral surface of the medulla (Figure 8-2).

The central chemoreceptors are surrounded by brain extracellular fluid and respond to changes in its H^+ concentration. An increase in H^+ concentration stimulates ventilation, whereas a decrease inhibits it. The composition of the extracellular fluid around the receptors is governed by the cerebrospinal fluid (CSF), local blood flow, and local metabolism.

Of these, the CSF is apparently the most important. It is separated from the blood by the blood-brain barrier, which is relatively impermeable to H^+ and HCO_3^- ions, although molecular CO_2 diffuses across it easily. When the blood Pco_2 rises, CO_2 diffuses into the CSF from the cerebral blood vessels, liberating H^+ ions that stimulate the chemoreceptors. Thus, the CO_2 level in blood regulates ventilation chiefly by its effect on the pH of the CSF. The resulting hyperventilation reduces the Pco_2 in the blood and therefore in the

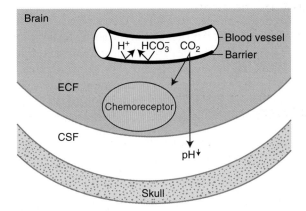

Figure 8-2. Environment of the central chemoreceptors. They are bathed in brain extracellular fluid (ECF), through which CO_2 easily diffuses from blood vessels to cerebrospinal fluid (CSF). The CO_2 reduces the CSF pH, thus stimulating the chemoreceptor. H^+ and HCO_3^- ions cannot easily cross the blood-brain barrier.

CSF. The cerebral vasodilation that accompanies an increased arterial P_{CO_2} enhances diffusion of CO_2 into the CSF and the brain extracellular fluid.

The normal pH of the CSF is 7.32, and because the CSF contains much less protein than blood, it has a much lower buffering capacity. As a result, the change in CSF pH for a given change in P_{CO_2} is greater than in blood. If the CSF pH is displaced over a prolonged period, a compensatory change in HCO_3^-. occurs as a result of transport across the blood-brain barrier. However, the CSF pH does not usually return all the way to 7.32. The change in CSF pH occurs more promptly than the change of the pH of arterial blood by renal compensation (Figure 6-8), a process that takes 2 to 3 days. Because CSF pH returns to near its normal value more rapidly than does blood pH, CSF pH has a more important effect on changes in the level of ventilation and the arterial P_{CO_2}.

One example of these changes is a patient with chronic lung disease and CO_2 retention of long standing who may have a nearly normal CSF pH and, therefore, an abnormally low ventilation for his or her arterial P_{CO_2}. A similar situation is seen in normal subjects who are exposed to an atmosphere containing 3% CO_2 for some days.

Central Chemoreceptors

- Located near the ventral surface of the medulla
- Sensitive to the P_{CO_2} but not P_{O_2} of blood
- Respond to the change in pH of the ECF/CSF when CO_2 diffuses out of cerebral capillaries

Peripheral Chemoreceptors

Peripheral chemoreceptors are located in the carotid bodies at the bifurcation of the common carotid arteries, and in the aortic bodies above and below the aortic arch. The carotid bodies are the most important in humans. They contain glomus cells of two types. Type I cells show an intense fluorescent staining because of their large content of dopamine. These cells are in close apposition to endings of the afferent carotid sinus nerve (Figure 8-3). The carotid body also contains type II cells and a rich supply of capillaries. The precise mechanism of the carotid bodies is still uncertain, but many physiologists believe that the glomus cells are the sites of chemoreception and that modulation of neurotransmitter release from the glomus cells by physiological and chemical stimuli affects the discharge rate of the carotid body afferent fibers (Figure 8-3A).

The peripheral chemoreceptors respond to decreases in arterial P_{O_2} and pH, and increases in arterial P_{CO_2}. They are unique among tissues of the body in that their sensitivity to changes in arterial P_{O_2} begins around 500 mm Hg. Figure 8-3B shows that the relationship between firing rate and

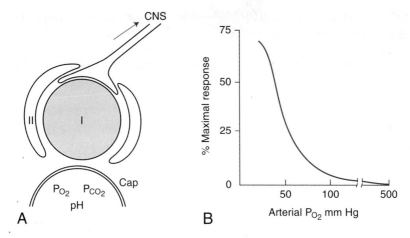

Figure 8-3. A. Diagram of a carotid body that contains type I and type II cells with many capillaries (Cap). Impulses travel to the central nervous system (CNS) through the carotid sinus nerve. **B** shows the nonlinear response to arterial P_{O_2}. Note that the maximum response occurs below a P_{O_2} of 50 mm Hg.

arterial P_{O_2} is very nonlinear; relatively little response occurs until the arterial P_{O_2} is reduced below 100 mm Hg, but then the rate rapidly increases. The carotid bodies have a very high blood flow for their size, and therefore, in spite of their high metabolic rate, the arterial-venous O_2 difference is small. As a result, they respond to arterial rather than to venous P_{O_2}. The response of these receptors can be very fast; indeed, their discharge rate can alter during the respiratory cycle as a result of the small cyclic changes in blood gases. The peripheral chemoreceptors are responsible for all the increase of ventilation that occurs in humans in response to arterial hypoxemia. Indeed, in the absence of these receptors, severe hypoxemia may depress ventilation, presumably through a direct effect on the respiratory centers. Complete loss of hypoxic ventilatory drive has been shown in patients with bilateral carotid body resection.

The response of the peripheral chemoreceptors to arterial P_{CO_2} is less important than that of the central chemoreceptors. For example, when a normal subject is given a CO_2 mixture to breathe, less than 20% of the ventilatory response can be attributed to the peripheral chemoreceptors. However, their response is more rapid, and they may be useful in matching ventilation to abrupt changes in P_{CO_2}.

In humans, the carotid but not the aortic bodies respond to a fall in arterial pH. This occurs regardless of whether the cause is respiratory or metabolic. Interaction of the various stimuli occurs. Thus, increases in chemoreceptor activity in response to decreases in arterial P_{O_2} are potentiated by increases in P_{CO_2} and, in the carotid bodies, by decreases in pH.

Peripheral Chemoreceptors

- Located in the carotid and aortic bodies
- Respond to decreased arterial P_{O_2}, and increased P_{CO_2} and H^+
- Rapidly responding

Lung Receptors

1. Pulmonary Stretch Receptors

Pulmonary stretch receptors are also known as slowly adapting pulmonary stretch receptors and are believed to lie within airway smooth muscle. They discharge in response to distension of the lung, and their activity is sustained with lung inflation; that is, they show little adaptation. The impulses travel in the vagus nerve via large myelinated fibers.

The main reflex effect of stimulating these receptors is a slowing of respiratory frequency due to an increase in expiratory time. This is known as the Hering-Breuer inflation reflex. It can be well demonstrated in a rabbit preparation in which the diaphragm contains a slip of muscle from which recordings can be made without interfering with the other respiratory muscles. Classic experiments showed that inflation of the lungs tended to inhibit further inspiratory muscle activity. The opposite response is also seen; that is, deflation of the lungs tends to initiate inspiratory activity (deflation reflex). Thus, these reflexes can provide a self-regulatory mechanism or negative feedback.

The Hering-Breuer reflexes were once thought to play a major role in ventilation by determining the rate and depth of breathing. This could be done by using the information from these stretch receptors to modulate the "switching-off" mechanism in the medulla. For example, bilateral vagotomy, which removes the input of these receptors, causes slow, deep breathing in most animals. However, more recent work indicates that the reflexes are largely inactive in adult humans unless the tidal volume exceeds 1 liter, as in exercise. Transient bilateral blockade of the vagi by local anesthesia in awake humans does not change either breathing rate or volume. There is some evidence that these reflexes may be more important in newborn babies.

2. Irritant Receptors

These are thought to lie between airway epithelial cells, and they are stimulated by noxious gases, cigarette smoke, inhaled dusts, and cold air. The impulses travel up the vagus in myelinated fibers, and the reflex effects include bronchoconstriction and hyperpnea. Some physiologists prefer to call these receptors "rapidly adapting pulmonary stretch receptors" because they show rapid adaptation and are apparently involved in additional mechanoreceptor functions, as well as responding to noxious stimuli on the airway walls.

It is possible that irritant receptors play a role in the bronchoconstriction of asthma attacks as a result of their response to released histamine.

3. J Receptors

These are the endings of nonmyelinated C fibers and sometimes go by this name. The term "juxtacapillary," or J, is used because these receptors are believed to be in the alveolar walls, close to the capillaries. The evidence for this location is that they respond very quickly to chemicals injected into the pulmonary circulation. The impulses pass up the vagus nerve in slowly conducting nonmyelinated fibers and can result in rapid, shallow breathing, although intense stimulation causes apnea. There is evidence that engorgement of pulmonary capillaries and increases in the interstitial fluid volume of the alveolar wall activate these receptors. They may play a role in the rapid, shallow breathing and dyspnea (sensation of difficulty in breathing) associated with left heart failure and interstitial lung disease.

4. Bronchial C Fibers

These are supplied by the bronchial circulation rather than the pulmonary circulation as is the case for the J receptors described above. They respond quickly to chemicals injected into the bronchial circulation. The reflex responses to stimulation include rapid shallow breathing, bronchoconstriction, and mucous secretion.

Other Receptors

1. Nose and Upper Airway Receptors

The nose, nasopharynx, larynx, and trachea contain receptors that respond to mechanical and chemical stimulation. These are an extension of the irritant receptors described above. Various reflex responses have been described, including sneezing, coughing, and bronchoconstriction. Laryngeal spasm may occur if the larynx is irritated mechanically, for example, during insertion of an endotracheal tube with insufficient local anesthesia.

2. Joint and Muscle Receptors

Impulses from moving limbs are believed to be part of the stimulus to ventilation during exercise, especially in the early stages.

3. Gamma System

Many muscles, including the intercostal muscles and diaphragm, contain muscle spindles that sense elongation of the muscle. This information is used to reflexly control the strength of contraction. These receptors may be involved in the sensation of dyspnea that occurs when unusually large respiratory efforts are required to move the lung and chest wall, for example, because of airway obstruction.

4. Arterial Baroreceptors

An increase in arterial blood pressure can cause reflex hypoventilation or apnea through stimulation of the aortic and carotid sinus baroreceptors. Conversely, a decrease in blood pressure may result in hyperventilation.

5. Pain and Temperature

Stimulation of many afferent nerves can bring about changes in ventilation. Pain often causes a period of apnea followed by hyperventilation. Heating of the skin may result in hyperventilation.

▶ Integrated Responses

Now that we have looked at the various units that make up the respiratory control system (Figure 8-1), it is useful to consider the overall responses of the system to changes in the arterial CO_2, O_2, and pH and to exercise.

Response to Carbon Dioxide

The most important factor in the control of ventilation under normal conditions is the Pco_2 of the arterial blood. The sensitivity of this control is remarkable. In the course of daily activity with periods of rest and exercise, the arterial Pco_2 is probably held to within 3 mm Hg. During sleep, it may rise a little more.

The ventilatory response to CO_2 is normally measured by having the subject inhale CO_2 mixtures or rebreathe from a bag so that the inspired Pco_2 gradually rises. In one technique, the subject rebreathes from a bag that is prefilled with 7% CO_2 and 93% O_2. As the subject rebreathes, metabolic CO_2 is added to the bag, but the O_2 concentration remains relatively high. In such a procedure, the Pco_2 of the bag gas increases at the rate of about 4 mm Hg·min⁻¹.

Figure 8-4 shows the results of experiments in which the inspired mixture was adjusted to yield a constant alveolar Po_2. (In this type of experiment on normal subjects, alveolar end-tidal Po_2 and Pco_2 are generally taken to reflect the arterial levels.) It can be seen that with a normal Po_2 the ventilation increases by about 2 to 3 liters·min⁻¹ for each 1 mm Hg rise in Pco_2. Lowering the Po_2 produces two effects: ventilation for a given Pco_2 is higher, and the slope of the line becomes steeper. There is considerable variation between subjects.

Another way of measuring respiratory drive is to record the inspiratory pressure during a brief period of airway occlusion. The subject breathes through a mouthpiece attached to a valve box, and the inspiratory port is provided with a shutter. This is closed during an expiration (the subject being unaware), so that the first part of the next inspiration is against an occluded

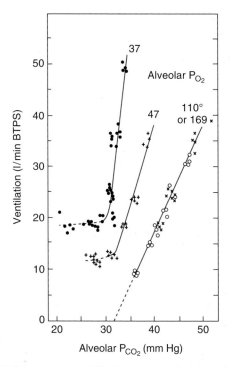

Figure 8-4. Ventilatory response to CO_2. Each curve of total ventilation against alveolar P_{CO_2} is for a different alveolar P_{O_2}. In this study, no difference was found between alveolar P_{O_2} values of 110 mm Hg and 169 mm Hg, though some investigators have found that the slope of the line is slightly less at the higher P_{O_2}.

airway. The shutter is opened after about 0.5 second. The pressure generated during the first 0.1 second of attempted inspiration (known as $P_{0.1}$) is taken as a measure of respiratory center output. This is largely unaffected by the mechanical properties of the respiratory system, although it is influenced by lung volume. This method can be used to study the respiratory sensitivity to CO_2, hypoxia, and other variables as well.

Ventilatory Response to Carbon Dioxide

- Arterial P_{CO_2} is the most important stimulus to ventilation under most conditions and is normally tightly controlled
- Most of the stimulus comes from the central chemoreceptors, but the peripheral chemoreceptors also contribute and their response is faster
- The response is magnified if the arterial P_{O_2} is lowered

A reduction in arterial P_{CO_2} is very effective in reducing the stimulus to ventilation. For example, if the reader hyperventilates voluntarily for a few seconds, he or she will find that there is no urge to breathe for a short period. An anesthetized patient will frequently stop breathing for a minute or so if first overventilated by the anesthesiologist.

The ventilatory response to CO_2 is reduced by sleep, increasing age, and genetic, racial, and personality factors. Trained athletes and divers tend to have a low CO_2 sensitivity. Various drugs depress the respiratory center, including morphine and barbiturates. Patients who have taken an overdose of one of these drugs often have marked hypoventilation. The ventilatory response to CO_2 is also reduced if the work of breathing is increased. This can be demonstrated by having normal subjects breathe through a narrow tube. The neural output of the respiratory center is not reduced, but it is not so effective in producing ventilation. The abnormally small ventilatory response to CO_2 and the CO_2 retention in some patients with lung disease can be partly explained by the same mechanism. In such patients, reducing the airway resistance with bronchodilators often increases their ventilatory response. There is also some evidence that the sensitivity of the respiratory center is reduced in these patients.

As we have seen, the main stimulus to increase ventilation when the arterial P_{CO_2} rises comes from the central chemoreceptors, which respond to the increased H^+ concentration of the brain extracellular fluid near the receptors. An additional stimulus comes from the peripheral chemoreceptors, because of both the rise in arterial P_{CO_2} and the fall in pH.

Response to Oxygen

The way in which a reduction of P_{O_2} in arterial blood stimulates ventilation can be studied by having a subject breathe hypoxic gas mixtures. The end-tidal

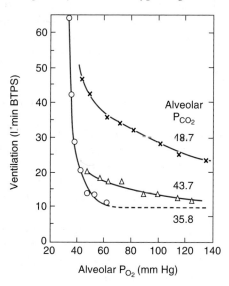

Figure 8-5. Hypoxic response curves. Note that when the P_{CO_2} is 35.8 mm Hg, almost no increase in ventilation occurs until the P_{O_2} is reduced to about 50 mm Hg.

Po_2 and Pco_2 are used as a measure of the arterial values. Figure 8-5 shows that when the alveolar Pco_2 is kept at about 36 mm Hg (by altering the inspired mixture), the alveolar Po_2 can be reduced to the vicinity of 50 mm Hg before any appreciable increase in ventilation occurs. Raising the Pco_2 increases the ventilation at any Po_2 (compare Figure 8-4). Note that when the Pco_2 is increased, a reduction in Po_2 below 100 mm Hg causes some stimulation of ventilation, unlike the situation in which the Pco_2 is normal. Thus, the combined effects of both stimuli exceed the sum of each stimulus given separately; this is referred to as interaction between the high CO_2 and low O_2 stimuli. Large differences in response occur between individual subjects.

Because the Po_2 can normally be reduced so far without evoking a ventilatory response, the role of this hypoxic stimulus in the day-to-day control of ventilation is small. However, on ascent to high altitude, a large increase in ventilation occurs in response to the hypoxia (see Chapter 9).

In some patients with severe lung disease, the hypoxic drive to ventilation becomes very important. These patients have chronic CO_2 retention, and the pH of their brain extracellular fluid has returned to near normal in spite of a raised Pco_2. Thus, they have lost most of their increase in the stimulus to ventilation from CO_2. In addition, the initial depression of blood pH has been nearly abolished by renal compensation, so there is little pH stimulation of the peripheral chemoreceptors (see below). Under these conditions, the arterial hypoxemia becomes the chief stimulus to ventilation. If such a patient is given a high O_2 mixture to breathe to relieve the hypoxemia, ventilation may become grossly depressed. The ventilatory state is best monitored by measuring arterial Pco_2.

As we have seen, hypoxemia reflexly stimulates ventilation by its action on the carotid and aortic body chemoreceptors. It has no action on the central chemoreceptors; indeed, in the absence of peripheral chemoreceptors, hypoxemia depresses respiration. However, prolonged hypoxemia can cause mild cerebral acidosis, which, in turn, can stimulate ventilation.

Response to pH

A reduction in arterial blood pH stimulates ventilation. In practice, it is often difficult to separate the ventilatory response resulting from a fall in pH from that caused by an accompanying rise in Pco_2. However, in experimental animals in which it is possible to reduce the pH at a constant Pco_2, the stimulus to ventilation can be convincingly demonstrated. Patients with a partly compensated metabolic acidosis (such as uncontrolled diabetes mellitus) who have a low pH and low Pco_2 (Figure 6-8) show an increased ventilation. Indeed, this is responsible for the reduced Pco_2.

As we have seen, the chief site of action of a reduced arterial pH is the peripheral chemoreceptors. It is also possible that the central chemoreceptors or the respiratory center itself can be affected by a change in blood pH if it is large enough. In this case, the blood-brain barrier becomes partly permeable to H^+ ions.

Ventilatory Response to Hypoxia

- Only the peripheral chemoreceptors are involved
- There is negligible control during normoxic conditions
- The control becomes important at high altitude and in long-term hypoxemia caused by chronic lung disease

---

Response to Exercise

On exercise, ventilation increases promptly and during strenuous exertion may reach very high levels. Fit young people who attain a maximum O_2 consumption of 4 liters·min^{-1} may have a total ventilation of 120 liters·min^{-1}, that is, about 15 times their resting level. This increase in ventilation closely matches the increase in O_2 uptake and CO_2 output. It is remarkable that the cause of the increased ventilation on exercise remains largely unknown.

The arterial Pco_2 does not increase during exercise; indeed, during severe exercise, it typically falls slightly. The arterial Po_2 usually increases slightly, although it may fall at very high work levels. The arterial pH remains nearly constant for moderate exercise, although during heavy exercise it falls because of the liberation of lactic acid through anaerobic glycolysis. It is clear, therefore, that none of the mechanisms we have discussed so far can account for the large increase in ventilation observed during light to moderate exercise.

Other stimuli have been suggested. Passive movement of the limbs stimulates ventilation in both anesthetized animals and awake humans. This is a reflex with receptors presumably located in joints or muscles. It may be responsible for the abrupt increase in ventilation that occurs during the first few seconds of exercise. One hypothesis is that *oscillations in arterial Po_2 and Pco_2* may stimulate the peripheral chemoreceptors, even though the mean level remains unaltered. These fluctuations are caused by the periodic nature of ventilation and increase when the tidal volume rises, as on exercise. Another theory is that the central chemoreceptors increase ventilation to hold the *arterial Pco_2 constant* by some kind of servomechanism, just as the thermostat can control a furnace with little change in temperature. The objection that the arterial Pco_2 often *falls* on exercise is countered by the assertion that the preferred level of Pco_2 is reset in some way. Proponents of this theory believe that the ventilatory response to inhaled CO_2 may not be a reliable guide to what happens on exercise.

Yet another hypothesis is that ventilation is linked in some way to the additional CO_2 *load* presented to the lungs in the mixed venous blood during exercise. In animal experiments, an increase in this load produced either by infusing CO_2 into the venous blood or by increasing venous return has been shown to correlate well with ventilation. However, a problem with this hypothesis is that no suitable receptor has been found.

Additional factors that have been suggested include the *increase in body temperature* during exercise, which stimulates ventilation, and *impulses from the motor cortex.* However, none of the theories proposed so far is completely satisfactory.

▶ Abnormal Patterns of Breathing

Subjects with severe hypoxemia often exhibit a striking pattern of periodic breathing known as *Cheyne-Stokes respiration.* This is characterized by periods of apnea of 10 to 20 seconds, separated by approximately equal periods of hyperventilation when the tidal volume gradually waxes and then wanes. This pattern is frequently seen at high altitude, especially at night during sleep. It is also found in some patients with severe heart disease or brain damage.

The pattern can be reproduced in experimental animals by lengthening the distance through which blood travels on its way to the brain from the lung. Under these conditions, there is a long delay before the central chemoreceptors sense the alteration in P_{CO_2} caused by a change in ventilation. As a result, the respiratory center hunts for the equilibrium condition, always overshooting it. However, not all instances of Cheyne-Stokes respiration can be explained on this basis. Other abnormal patterns of breathing can also occur in disease.

KEY CONCEPTS

1. The respiratory centers that are responsible for the rhythmic pattern of breathing are located in the pons and medulla of the brainstem. The output of these centers can be overridden by the cortex to some extent.
2. The central chemoreceptors are located near the ventral surface of the medulla and respond to changes in pH of the CSF, which in turn are caused by diffusion of CO_2 from brain capillaries. Alterations in the bicarbonate concentration of the CSF modulate the pH and therefore the chemoreceptor response.
3. The peripheral chemoreceptors, chiefly in the carotid bodies, respond to a reduced P_{O_2} and increases in P_{CO_2} and H^+ concentration. The response to O_2 is small above a P_{O_2} of 50 mm Hg. The response to increased CO_2 is less marked than that from the central chemoreceptors but occurs more rapidly.
4. Other receptors are located in the walls of the airways and alveoli.
5. The P_{CO_2} of the blood is the most important factor controlling ventilation under normal conditions, and most of the control is via the central chemoreceptors.
6. The P_{O_2} of the blood does not normally affect ventilation, but it becomes important at high altitude and in some patients with lung disease.
7. Exercise causes a large increase in ventilation, but the cause, especially during moderate exercise, is poorly understood.

QUESTIONS

For each question, choose the one best answer.

1. Concerning the respiratory centers,

   A. The normal rhythmic pattern of breathing originates from neurons in the motor area of the cortex.

B. During quiet breathing, expiratory neurons fire actively.
C. Impulses from the pneumotaxic center can stimulate inspiratory activity.
D. The cortex of the brain can override the function of the respiratory centers.
E. The only output from the respiratory centers is via the phrenic nerves.

2. Concerning the central chemoreceptors,

A. They are located near the dorsal surface of the medulla.
B. They respond to both the P_{CO_2} and the P_{O_2} of the blood.
C. They are activated by changes in the pH of the surrounding extracellular fluid.
D. For a given rise in P_{CO_2}, the pH of cerebrospinal fluid falls less than that of blood.
E. The bicarbonate concentration of the CSF cannot affect their output.

3. Concerning the peripheral chemoreceptors,

A. They respond to changes in the arterial P_{O_2} but not pH.
B. Under normoxic conditions, the response to changes in P_{O_2} is very small.
C. The response to changes in P_{CO_2} is slower than for central chemoreceptors.
D. They are the most important receptors causing an increased ventilation in response to a rise in P_{CO_2}.
E. They have a low blood flow per gram of tissue.

4. Concerning the ventilatory response to carbon dioxide,

A. It is increased if the alveolar P_{O_2} is raised.
B. It depends only on the central chemoreceptors.
C. It is increased during sleep.
D. It is increased if the work of breathing is raised.
E. It is a major factor controlling the normal level of ventilation.

5. Concerning the ventilatory response to hypoxia,

A. It is the major stimulus to ventilation at high altitude.
B. It is primarily brought about by the central chemoreceptors.
C. It is reduced if the P_{CO_2} is also raised.
D. It rarely stimulates ventilation in patients with chronic lung disease.
E. It is important in mild carbon monoxide poisoning.

6. The most important stimulus controlling the level of resting ventilation is

A. P_{O_2} on peripheral chemoreceptors.
B. P_{CO_2} on peripheral chemoreceptors.
C. pH on peripheral chemoreceptors.
D. pH of CSF on central chemoreceptors.
E. P_{O_2} on central chemoreceptors.

7. Exercise is one of the most powerful stimulants to ventilation. It primarily works by way of

A. Low arterial P_{O_2}.
B. High arterial P_{CO_2}.
C. Low P_{O_2} in mixed venous blood.
D. Low arterial pH.
E. None of the above.

8. Concerning the Hering-Breuer inflation reflex,

A. The impulses travel to the brain via the carotid sinus nerve.
B. It results in further inspiratory efforts if the lung is maintained inflated.
C. It is seen in adults at small tidal volumes.
D. It may help to inflate the newborn lung.
E. Abolishing the reflex in many animals causes rapid, shallow breathing.

Respiratory System Under Stress

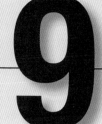

▶ HOW GAS EXCHANGE
IS ACCOMPLISHED
DURING EXERCISE,
AT LOW AND HIGH
PRESSURES, AND AT
BIRTH

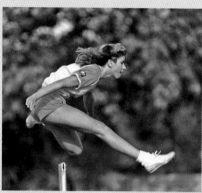

The normal lung has enormous reserves at rest, and these enable it to meet the greatly increased demands for gas exchange during exercise. In addition, the lung serves as our principal physiological link with the environment in which we live; its surface area is some 30 times greater than that of the skin. The human urge to climb higher and dive deeper puts the respiratory system under great stress, although these situations are minor insults compared with the process of being born!

▶ Exercise

The gas exchange demands of the lung are enormously increased by exercise. Typically, the resting oxygen consumptions of 300 ml·min^{-1} can rise to about 3000 ml·min^{-1} in a moderately fit subject (and as high as 6000 ml·min^{-1} in an elite athlete). Similarly, the resting CO_2 output of, say, 240 ml·min^{-1} increases to about 3000 ml·min^{-1}. Typically, the respiratory exchange ratio (R) rises from about 0.8 at rest to 1.0 on exercise. This increase reflects a greater reliance on carbohydrate rather than fat to produce the required energy. Indeed, R often reaches even higher levels during the unsteady state of severe exercise when lactic acid is produced by anaerobic glycolysis, and additional CO_2 is therefore eliminated from bicarbonate. In addition, there is increased CO_2 elimination because the increased H^+ concentration stimulates the peripheral chemoreceptors, thus increasing ventilation.

Exercise is conveniently studied on a treadmill or stationary bicycle. As work rate (or power) is increased, oxygen uptake increases linearly (Figure 9-1A). However, above a certain work rate, $\dot{V}o_2$ becomes constant; this is known as the $\dot{V}o_2$ max. An increase in work rate above this level can occur only through anaerobc glycolysis.

Ventilation also increases linearly initially when plotted against work rate or $\dot{V}o_2$, but at high $\dot{V}o_2$ values, it increases more rapidly because lactic acid is liberated, and this increases the ventilatory stimulus (Figure 9-1B). Sometimes there is a clear break in the slope; this has been called the *anaerobic threshold* or *ventilation threshold* although the term is somewhat controversial. Unfit subjects produce lactate at relatively low work levels, whereas well-trained subjects can reach fairly high work levels before substantial anaerobic glycolysis occurs.

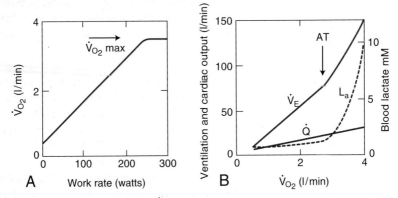

Figure 9-1. A. O_2 consumption ($\dot{V}o_2$) increases nearly linearly with work rate until the $\dot{V}o_2$ max is reached. **B.** Ventilation initially increases linearly with O_2 consumption but rises more rapidly when substantial amounts of blood lactate are formed. If there is a clear break, this is sometimes called the anaerobic or ventilation threshold (AT). Cardiac output increases more slowly than ventilation.

Many functions of the respiratory system change in response to exercise. The diffusing capacity of the lung increases because of increases in both the diffusing capacity of the membrane, D_M and the volume of blood in the pulmonary capillaries, V_c. These changes are brought about by recruitment and distension of pulmonary capillaries, particularly in the upper parts of the lung. Typically, the diffusing capacity increases at least threefold. Nevertheless, some elite athletes at extremely high work levels show a fall in arterial Po_2 caused by diffusion limitation because of the reduced time available for the loading of oxygen in the pulmonary capillary (Figure 3-3).

Cardiac output increases approximately linearly with work level as a result of increases in both heart rate and stroke volume. However, the change in cardiac output is only about a quarter of the increase in ventilation (in liter·min^{-1}). This makes sense because it is much easier to move air than to move blood. If we look at the Fick equation, $\dot{V}_{O_2} = Q(Ca_{O_2} - C_{\bar{V}_{O_2}})$, the increase in $\dot{V}_{O_2}$ is brought about by both an increase in cardiac output and a rise in arterial-venous O_2 difference because of the fall in the oxygen concentration of mixed venous blood. By contrast, if we look at the analogous equation for ventilation, $\dot{V}_{O_2} = \dot{V}_E(F_{I_{O_2}} - F_{E_{O_2}})$, the difference between inspired and expired O_2 concentrations does not change. This is consistent with the much larger increase in ventilation than blood flow. The increase in cardiac output is associated with elevations of both the pulmonary arterial and pulmonary venous pressures, which account for the recruitment and distension of pulmonary capillaries. Pulmonary vascular resistance falls.

In normal subjects, the amount of ventilation-perfusion inequality decreases during moderate exercise because of the more uniform topographical distribution of blood flow. However, because the degree of ventilation-perfusion inequality in normal subjects is trivial, this is of little consequence. There is some evidence that in elite athletes at very high work levels, some ventilation-perfusion inequality develops, possibly because of mild degrees of interstitial pulmonary edema. Certainly, fluid must move out of pulmonary capillaries because of the increased pressure within them.

The oxygen dissociation curve moves to the right in exercising muscles because of the increase in Pco_2, H^+ concentration, and temperature. This assists the unloading of oxygen to the muscles. When the blood returns to the lung, the temperature of the blood falls a little and the curve shifts leftward somewhat. In some animals, such as horses and dogs, the hematocrit increases on exercise because red cells are ejected from the spleen, but this does not occur in humans.

In peripheral tissues, additional capillaries open up, thus reducing the diffusion path length to the mitochondria. Peripheral vascular resistance falls because the large increase in cardiac output is not associated with much of an increase in mean arterial pressure, at least during dynamic exercise such as running. During static exercise such as weight lifting, large increases in systemic arterial pressure often occur. Exercise training increases the number of capillaries and mitochondria in skeletal muscle.

As we saw in Chapter 8, the very large increase in ventilation that occurs during exercise is largely unexplained. However, the net result is that the arterial P_{O_2}, P_{CO_2}, and pH are little affected by moderate exercise. At very high work levels, P_{CO_2} often falls, P_{O_2} rises, and pH falls because of lactic acidosis.

▶ High Altitude

The barometric pressure decreases with distance above the earth's surface in an approximately exponential manner (Figure 9-2). The pressure at 5800 m (19,000 ft) is only one-half the normal 760 mm Hg, so the P_{O_2} of moist inspired gas is $(380 - 47) \times 0.2093 = 70$ mm Hg (47 mm Hg is the partial pressure of water vapor at body temperature). At the summit of Mount Everest (altitude 8848 m, or 29,028 ft), the inspired P_{O_2} is only 43 mm Hg. At 19,200 m (63,000 ft), the barometric pressure is 47 mm Hg, so the inspired P_{O_2} is zero.

In spite of the hypoxia associated with high altitude, some 140 million people live at elevations over 2500 m (8000 ft), and permanent residents live higher than 5000 m (16,400 ft) in the Andes. A remarkable degree of acclimatization occurs when humans ascend to these altitudes; indeed, climbers have lived for several days at altitudes that would cause unconsciousness within a few seconds in the absence of acclimatization.

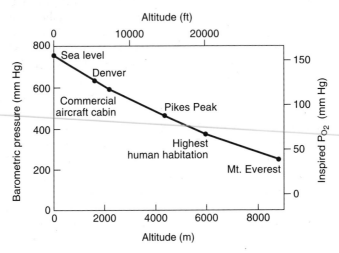

Figure 9-2. Relationship between altitude and barometric pressure. Note that the P_{O_2} of moist inspired gas is about 130 mm Hg at 1520 m (5000 ft) (Denver, CO) but is only 43 mm Hg on the summit of Mount Everest.

Hyperventilation

The most important feature of acclimatization to high altitude is hyperventilation. Its physiological value can be seen by considering the alveolar gas equation for a climber on the summit of Mount Everest. If the climber's alveolar P_{CO_2} was 40 and respiratory exchange ratio 1, the climber's alveolar P_{O_2} would be 43 – (40/1)* = 3 mm Hg! However, by increasing the climber's ventilation fivefold, and thus reducing the P_{CO_2} to 8 mm Hg (see p. 20), the alveolar P_{O_2} is increased to 43 – 8 = 35 mm Hg. Typically, the arterial P_{CO_2} in permanent residents at 4600 m (15,000 ft) is about 33 mm Hg.

The mechanism of the hyperventilation is hypoxic stimulation of the peripheral chemoreceptors. The resulting low arterial P_{CO_2} and alkalosis tend to inhibit this increase in ventilation, but after a day or so, the cerebrospinal fluid (CSF) pH is brought partly back by movement of bicarbonate out of the CSF, and after 2 or 3 days, the pH of the arterial blood is returned nearer to normal by renal excretion of bicarbonate. These brakes on ventilation are then reduced, and it increases further. In addition, there is now evidence that the sensitivity of the carotid bodies to hypoxia increases during acclimatization. Interestingly, people who are born at high altitude have a diminished ventilatory response to hypoxia that is only slowly corrected by subsequent residence at sea level.

Polycythemia

Another apparently valuable feature of acclimatization to high altitude is an increase in the red blood cell concentration of the blood. The resulting rise in hemoglobin concentration, and therefore O_2-carrying capacity, means that although the arterial P_{O_2} and O_2 saturation are diminished, the O_2 concentration of the arterial blood may be normal or even above normal. For example, in some permanent residents at 4600 m (15,000 ft) in the Peruvian Andes, the arterial P_{O_2} is only 45 mm Hg, and the corresponding arterial O_2 saturation is only 81%. Ordinarily, this would considerably decrease the arterial O_2 concentration, but because of the polycythemia, the hemoglobin concentration is increased from 15 to 19.8 g/100 ml, giving an arterial O_2 concentration of 22.4 ml/100 ml, which is actually higher than the normal sea level value. The polycythemia also tends to maintain the P_{O_2} of mixed venous blood, and typically in Andean natives living at 4600 m (15,000 ft), this P_{O_2} is only 7 mm Hg below normal (Figure 9-3). The stimulus for the increased production of red blood cells is hypoxemia, which releases erythropoietin from the kidney, which in turn stimulates the bone marrow. Polycythemia is also seen in many patients with chronic hypoxemia caused by lung or heart disease.

---

*When R = 1, the correction factor shown on p. 62 vanishes.

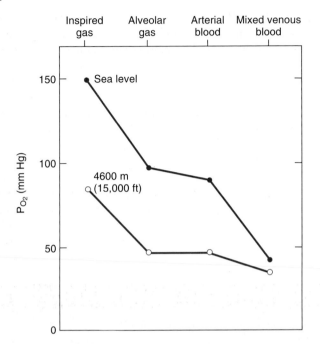

Figure 9-3. P_{O_2} values from inspired air to mixed venous blood at sea level and in residents at an altitude of 4600 m (15,000 ft). Note that in spite of the much lower inspired P_{O_2} at altitude, the P_{O_2} of the mixed venous blood is only 7 mm Hg lower.

Although the polycythemia of high altitude increases the O_2-carrying capacity of the blood, it also raises the blood viscosity. This can be deleterious, and some physiologists believe that the marked polycythemia that is sometimes seen is an inappropriate response.

Other Physiological Changes at High Altitude

There is a rightward shift of the O_2 dissociation curve at moderate altitudes that results in a better unloading of O_2 in venous blood at a given P_{O_2}. The cause of the shift is an increase in concentration of 2,3-diphosphoglycerate, which develops primarily because of the respiratory alkalosis. At higher altitudes, there is a *leftward shift* in the dissociation curve caused by the respiratory alkalosis, and this assists in the loading of O_2 in the pulmonary capillaries. The *number of capillaries per unit volume* in peripheral tissues increases, and changes occur in the *oxidative enzymes* inside the cells. The *maximum breathing capacity* increases because the air is less dense, and this assists the very high ventilations (up to 200 liters·min^{-1}) that occur on exercise. However, the maximum O_2 uptake declines rapidly above 4600 m (15,000 ft).

Pulmonary vasoconstriction occurs in response to alveolar hypoxia (Figure 4-10). This increases the pulmonary arterial pressure and the work done by the right heart. The hypertension is exaggerated by the polycythemia, which raises the viscosity of the blood. Hypertrophy of the right heart is seen, with characteristic changes in the electrocardiogram. There is no physiological advantage in this response, except that the topographical distribution of blood flow becomes more uniform. The pulmonary hypertension is sometimes associated with pulmonary edema, although the pulmonary venous pressure is normal. The probable mechanism is that the arteriolar vasoconstriction is uneven, and leakage occurs in unprotected, damaged capillaries. The edema fluid has a high protein concentration, indicating that the permeability of the capillaries is increased.

Newcomers to high altitude frequently complain of headache, fatigue, dizziness, palpitations, insomnia, loss of appetite, and nausea. This is known as *acute mountain sickness* and is attributable to the hypoxemia and alkalosis. Long-term residents sometimes develop an ill-defined syndrome characterized by marked polycythemia, fatigue, reduced exercise tolerance, and severe hypoxemia. This is called *chronic mountain sickness.*

Acclimatization to High Altitude

- Most important feature is hyperventilation
- Polycythemia is slow to develop and of minor value
- Other features include increases in cellular oxidative enzymes and the concentration of capillaries in some tissues
- Hypoxic pulmonary vasoconstriction is not beneficial

Permanent Residents of High Altitude

In some parts of the world, notably Tibet and the South American Andes, large numbers of people have lived at high altitude for many generations. It is now known that Tibetans exhibit features of natural selection to the hypoxia of high altitude. For example, there are differences in birth weight, hemoglobin concentrations, and arterial oxygen saturation in infants and exercising adults compared with lowlanders who go to high altitude.

Recent studies show that Tibetans have developed differences in their genetic makeup. For example, the gene that encodes the hypoxia-inducible factor 2α (HIF-2α) is more frequent in Tibetans than Han Chinese. HIF-2α is a transcription factor that regulates many physiological responses to hypoxia.

▶ O$_2$ Toxicity

The usual problem is getting enough O$_2$ into the body, but it is possible to have too much. When high concentrations of O$_2$ are breathed for many hours, damage to the lung may occur. If guinea pigs are placed in 100% O_2 at atmospheric pressure for 48 hours, they develop pulmonary edema. The first pathological changes are seen in the endothelial cells of the pulmonary capillaries (see Figure 1-1). It is (perhaps fortunately) difficult to administer very high concentrations of O_2 to patients, but evidence of impaired gas exchange has been demonstrated after 30 hours of inhalation of 100% O_2. Normal volunteers who breathe 100% O_2 at atmospheric pressure for 24 hours complain of substernal distress that is aggravated by deep breathing, and they develop a diminution of vital capacity of 500 to 800 ml. This is probably caused by absorption atelectasis (see below).

Another hazard of breathing 100% O_2 is seen in premature infants who develop blindness because of retrolental fibroplasia, that is, fibrous tissue formation behind the lens. Here the mechanism is local vasoconstriction caused by the high Po_2 in the incubator, and it can be avoided if the arterial Po_2 is kept below 140 mm Hg.

Absorption Atelectasis

This is another danger of breathing 100% O_2. Suppose that an airway is obstructed by mucus (Figure 9-4). The total pressure in the trapped gas is close to 760 mm Hg (it may be a few mm Hg less as it is absorbed because of elastic forces in the lung). But the sum of the partial pressures in the venous

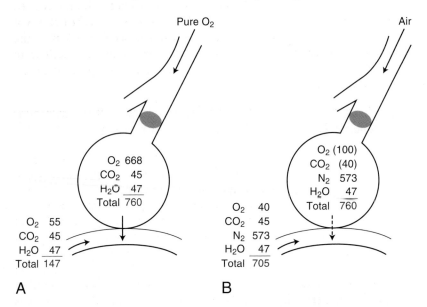

Figure 9-4. Reasons for atelectasis of alveoli beyond blocked airways when O_2 **(A)** and when air **(B)** is breathed. Note that in both cases, the sum of the gas partial pressures in the mixed venous blood is less than in the alveoli. In **(B)**, the Po_2 and Pco_2 are shown in *parentheses* because these values change with time. However, the total alveolar pressure remains within a few mm Hg of 760.

blood is far less than 760 mm Hg. This is because the P_{O_2} of the venous blood remains relatively low, even when O_2 is breathed. In fact, the rise in O_2 *concentration* of arterial and venous blood when O_2 is breathed will be the same if cardiac output remains unchanged, but because of the shape of the O_2 dissociation curve (see Figure 6-1), the increase in venous P_{O_2} is only about 10 to 15 mm Hg. Thus, because the sum of the partial pressures in the alveolar gas greatly exceeds that in the venous blood, gas diffuses into the blood, and rapid collapse of the alveoli occurs. Reopening such an atelectatic area may be difficult because of surface tension effects in such small units.

Absorption collapse also occurs in a blocked region even when air is breathed, although here the process is slower. Figure 9-4B shows that again the sum of the partial pressures in venous blood is less than 760 mm Hg because the fall in P_{O_2} from arterial to venous blood is much greater than the rise in P_{CO_2} (this is a reflection of the steeper slope of the CO_2 compared with the O_2 dissociation curve—see Figure 6-7). Because the total gas pressure in the alveoli is near 760 mm Hg, absorption is inevitable. Actually, the changes in the alveolar partial pressures during absorption are somewhat complicated, but it can be shown that the rate of collapse is limited by the rate of absorption of N_2. Because this gas has a low solubility, its presence acts as a "splint" that, as it were, supports the alveoli and delays collapse. Even relatively small concentrations of N_2 in alveolar gas have a useful splinting effect. Nevertheless, postoperative atelectasis is a common problem in patients who are treated with high O_2 mixtures. Collapse is particularly likely to occur at the bottom of the lung, where the parenchyma is least well expanded (see Figure 7-8) or the small airways are actually closed (see Figure 7-9). This same basic mechanism of absorption is responsible for the gradual disappearance of a pneumothorax, or a gas pocket introduced under the skin.

▶ Space Flight

The absence of gravity causes a number of physiological changes, and some of these affect the lung. The distribution of ventilation and blood flow become more uniform, with a small corresponding improvement in gas exchange (see Figures 5-8 and 5-10), though some inequality remains because of nongravitational factors. The deposition of inhaled aerosol is altered because of the absence of sedimentation. In addition, thoracic blood volume initially increases because blood does not pool in the legs, and this raises pulmonary capillary blood volume and diffusing capacity. Postural hypotension occurs on return to earth; this is known as *cardiovascular deconditioning*. Decalcification of bone, and muscle atrophy may occur, presumably through disuse. There is also a small reduction in red cell mass. Space sickness during the first few days of flight can be a serious operational problem.

▶ Increased Pressure

During diving, the pressure increases by 1 atm for every 10 m (33 ft) of descent. Pressure by itself is relatively innocuous, as long as it is balanced. However, if a gas cavity such as the lung, middle ear, or intracranial sinus fails to communicate with the outside, the pressure difference may cause compression on descent or overexpansion on ascent. For example, it is very important for scuba divers to exhale as they ascend to prevent overinflation and possible rupture of the lungs. The increased density of the gas at depth increases the work of breathing. This may result in CO_2 retention, especially on exercise.

Decompression Sickness

During diving, the high partial pressure of N_2 forces this poorly soluble gas into solution in body tissues. This particularly occurs in fat, which has a relatively high N_2 solubility. However, the blood supply of adipose tissue is meager, and the blood can carry little N_2. In addition, the gas diffuses slowly because of its low solubility. As a result, equilibration of N_2 between the tissues and the environment takes hours.

During ascent, N_2 is slowly removed from the tissues. If decompression is unduly rapid, bubbles of gaseous N_2 form, just as CO_2 is released when a bottle of champagne is opened. Some bubbles can occur without physiological disturbances, but large numbers of bubbles cause pain, especially in the region of joints ("bends"). In severe cases, there may be neurological disturbances such as deafness, impaired vision, and even paralysis caused by bubbles in the central nervous system (CNS) that obstruct blood flow.

The treatment of decompression sickness is by recompression. This reduces the volume of the bubbles and forces them back into solution, and often results in a dramatic reduction of symptoms. Prevention is by careful decompression in a series of regulated steps. Schedules, based partly on theory and partly on experience, exist that show how rapidly a diver can come up with little risk of developing bends. A short but very deep dive may require hours of gradual decompression. It is now known that bubble formation during ascent is very common. Therefore, the aim of the decompression schedules is to prevent the bubbles from growing too large.

Decompression Sickness

- Caused by the formation of N_2 bubbles during ascent from a deep dive
- May result in pain ("bends") and neurological disturbances
- Can be prevented by a slow, staged ascent
- Treated by recompression in a chamber
- Incidence is reduced by breathing a helium-oxygen mixture

The risk of decompression sickness following very deep dives can be reduced if a helium-O_2 mixture is breathed during the dive. Helium is about one-half as soluble as N_2, so less is dissolved in tissues. In addition, it has one-seventh of the molecular weight of N_2 and therefore diffuses out more rapidly through tissue (Figure 3-1). Both these factors reduce the risk of bends. Another advantage of a helium-O_2 mixture for divers is its low density, which reduces the work of breathing. Pure O_2 or enriched O_2 mixtures cannot be used at depth because of the dangers of O_2 toxicity (see below).

Commercial divers who are working at great depths, for example, on pipelines, sometimes use *saturation diving*. When they are not in the water, they live in a high-pressure chamber on the supply ship for several days, which means that they do not return to normal atmospheric pressure during this time. In this way they avoid decompression sickness. However, at the end of the period at high pressure, they may take many hours to decompress safely.

Inert Gas Narcosis

Although we usually think of N_2 as a physiological inert gas, at high partial pressures it affects the CNS. At a depth of about 50 m (160 ft), there is a feeling of euphoria (not unlike that following a martini or two), and scuba divers have been known to offer their mouthpieces to fish! At higher partial pressures, loss of coordination and eventually coma may develop.

The mechanism of action is not fully understood but may be related to the high fat-to-water solubility of N_2, which is a general property of anesthetic agents. Other gases, such as helium and hydrogen, can be used at much greater depths without narcotic effects.

O_2 Toxicity

We saw earlier that inhalation of 100% O_2 at 1 atm can damage the lung. Another form of O_2 toxicity is stimulation of the CNS, leading to convulsions, when the P_{O_2} considerably exceeds 760 mm Hg. The convulsions may be preceded by premonitory symptoms such as nausea, ringing in the ears, and twitching of the face.

The likelihood of convulsions depends on the inspired P_{O_2} and the duration of exposure, and it is increased if the subject is exercising. At a P_{O_2} of 4 atm, convulsions frequently occur within 30 minutes. For increasingly deep dives, the O_2 concentration is progressively reduced to avoid toxic effects and may eventually be less than 1% for a normal inspired P_{O_2}! The amateur scuba diver should *never* fill his or her tanks with O_2 because of the danger of a convulsion underwater. However, pure O_2 is sometimes used by the military for shallow dives because a closed breathing circuit with a CO_2 absorber leaves no telltale bubbles. The biochemical basis for the deleterious effects of a high P_{O_2} on the CNS is not fully understood but is probably the inactivation of certain enzymes, especially dehydrogenases containing sulfhydryl groups.

Hyperbaric O$_2$ Therapy

Increasing the arterial Po$_2$ to a very high level is useful in some clinical situations. One is severe CO poisoning in which most of the hemoglobin is bound to CO and is therefore unavailable to carry O$_2$. By raising the inspired Po$_2$ to 3 atm in special chambers, the amount of dissolved O$_2$ in arterial blood can be increased to about 6 ml/100 ml (see Figure 6-1), and thus the needs of the tissues can be met without functioning hemoglobin. Occasionally, an anemic crisis is managed in this way. Hyperbaric O$_2$ is also useful for treating gas gangrene because the organism cannot live in a high Po$_2$ environment. A hyperbaric chamber is also useful for treating decompression sickness.

Fire and explosions are serious hazards of a 100% O$_2$ atmosphere, especially at increased pressure. For this reason, O$_2$ in a pressure chamber is given by mask, and the chamber itself is filled with air.

▶ Polluted Atmospheres‡

Atmospheric pollution is an increasing problem in many countries as the number of motor vehicles and industries increases. The chief pollutants are various oxides of nitrogen and sulfur, ozone, carbon monoxide, various hydrocarbons, and particulate matter. Of these, nitrogen oxides, hydrocarbons, and CO are produced in large quantities by the internal combustion engine, the sulfur oxides mainly come from fossil fuel power stations, and ozone is chiefly formed in the atmosphere by the action of sunlight on nitrogen oxides and hydrocarbons. The concentration of atmospheric pollutants is greatly increased by a temperature inversion that prevents the normal escape of the warm surface air to the upper atmosphere.

Nitrogen oxides cause inflammation of the upper respiratory tract and eye irritation, and they are responsible for the yellow haze of smog. Sulfur oxides and ozone also cause bronchial inflammation, and ozone in high concentrations can produce pulmonary edema. The danger of CO is its propensity to tie up hemoglobin, and cyclic hydrocarbons are potentially carcinogenic. Both these pollutants exist in tobacco smoke, which is inhaled in far higher concentrations than any other atmospheric pollutant. There is evidence that some pollutants act synergistically, that is, their combined actions exceed the sum of their individual actions.

Many pollutants exist as *aerosols*, that is, very small particles that remain suspended in the air. When an aerosol is inhaled, its fate depends on the size of the particles. Large particles are removed by *impaction* in the nose and pharynx. This means that the particles are unable to turn the corners rapidly because of their inertia, and they impinge on the wet mucosa and are trapped. Medium-sized particles deposit in small airways and elsewhere because of their weight. This

‡For a more detailed account, see JB West, *Pulmonary Pathophysiology: The Essentials*, 7th ed. (Baltimore, MD: Lippincott Williams & Wilkins, 2007).

is called *sedimentation* and occurs especially where the flow velocity is suddenly reduced because of the enormous increase in combined airway cross section (Figure 1-5). For this reason, deposition is heavy in the terminal and respiratory bronchioles, and this region of a coal miner's lung shows a large dust concentration. The smallest particles (less than 0.1 μm in diameter) may reach the alveoli, where some deposition occurs through *diffusion* to the walls. Many small particles are not deposited at all but are exhaled with the next breath.

Once deposited, most of the particles are removed by various clearance mechanisms. Particles that deposit on bronchial walls are swept up the moving staircase of mucus that is propelled by cilia, and they are either swallowed or expectorated. However, the ciliary action can be paralyzed by inhaled irritants. Particles deposited in the alveoli are chiefly engulfed by macrophages that leave via the blood or lymphatics.

▶ Liquid Breathing

It is possible for mammals to survive for some hours breathing liquid instead of air. This was first shown with mice in saline in which the O_2 concentration was increased by exposure to 100% O_2 at 8 atm pressure. Subsequently, mice, rats, and dogs have survived a period of breathing fluorocarbon exposed to pure O_2 at 1 atm. This liquid has a high solubility for both O_2 and CO_2. The animals successfully returned to air breathing.

Because liquids have a much higher density and viscosity than air, the work of breathing is enormously increased. However, adequate oxygenation of the arterial blood can be obtained if the inspired concentration is raised sufficiently. Interestingly, a serious problem is eliminating CO_2. We saw earlier that diffusion within the airways is chiefly responsible for the gas exchange that occurs between the alveoli and the terminal or respiratory bronchioles, where bulk or convective flow takes over. Because the diffusion rates of gases in liquid are many orders of magnitude slower than in the gas phase, this means that a large partial pressure difference for CO_2 between alveoli and terminal bronchioles must be maintained. Animals breathing liquid, therefore, commonly develop CO_2 retention and acidosis. Note that the diffusion rate of O_2 can always be raised by increasing the inspired Po_2, but this option is not available to help eliminate CO_2.

▶ Perinatal Respiration

Placental Gas Exchange

During fetal life, gas exchange takes place through the placenta. Its circulation is in parallel with that of the peripheral tissues of the fetus (Figure 9-5), unlike the situation in the adult, in which the pulmonary circulation is in series with the systemic circulation. Maternal blood enters the placenta from the uterine arteries and surges into small spaces called intervillous sinusoids that function like the alveoli in the adult. Fetal blood from the aorta is supplied to capillary loops that protrude into the intervillous spaces. Gas exchange occurs across the blood-blood barrier, approximately 3.5 μm thick.

This arrangement is much less efficient for gas exchange than in the adult lung. Maternal blood apparently swirls around the sinusoids somewhat haphazardly, and there are probably large differences of Po_2 within these blood spaces. Contrast this situation with the air-filled alveoli, in which rapid gaseous diffusion stirs up the alveolar contents. The result is that the Po_2 of the fetal blood leaving the placenta is only about 30 mm Hg (Figure 9-5).

This blood mixes with venous blood draining from the fetal tissues and reaches the right atrium (RA) via the inferior vena cava. Because of streaming within the RA, most of this blood then flows directly into the left atrium (LA) through the open foramen ovale (FO) and thus is distributed via the ascending aorta to the brain and heart. Less-well-oxygenated blood returning to the RA via the superior vena cava finds its way to the right ventricle, but

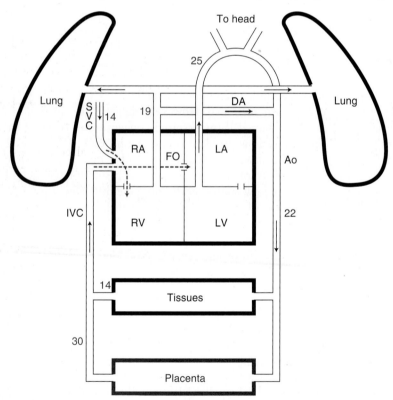

Figure 9-5. Blood circulation in the human fetus. The *numbers* show the approximate Po_2 of the blood in mm Hg. See text for details.

only a small portion reaches the lungs. Most is shunted to the aorta (Ao) through the ductus arteriosus (DA). The net result of this complex arrangement is that the best-oxygenated blood reaches the brain and heart, and the non–gas-exchanging lungs receive only about 15% of the cardiac output. Note that the arterial Po_2 in the descending aorta is only about 22 mm Hg.

To summarize the three most important differences between the fetal and adult circulations

1. The placenta is in parallel with the circulation to the tissues, whereas the lung is in series in the adult.

2. The DA shunts most of the blood from the pulmonary artery to the descending aorta.

3. Streaming within the RA means that the oxygenated blood from the placenta is preferentially delivered to the LA through the FO and therefore via the ascending aorta to the brain.

The First Breath

The emergence of a baby into the outside world is perhaps the most cataclysmic event of its life. The baby is suddenly bombarded with a variety of external stimuli. In addition, the process of birth interferes with placental gas exchange, with resulting hypoxemia and hypercapnia. Finally, the sensitivity of the chemoreceptors apparently increases dramatically at birth, although the mechanism is unknown. As a consequence of all these changes, the baby makes the first gasp.

The fetal lung is not collapsed but is inflated with liquid to about 40% of total lung capacity. This fluid is continuously secreted by alveolar cells during fetal life and has a low pH. Some of it is squeezed out as the infant moves through the birth canal, but the remainder helps in the subsequent inflation of the lung. As air enters the lung, large surface tension forces have to be overcome. Because the larger the radius of curvature, the lower the pressures (see Figure 7-4), this preinflation is believed to reduce the pressures required. Nevertheless, the intrapleural pressure during the first breath may fall to –40 cm water before any air enters the lung, and peak pressures as low as –100 cm water during the first few breaths have been recorded. These very large transient pressures are partly caused by the high viscosity of the lung liquid compared with air. The fetus makes very small, rapid breathing movements in the uterus over a considerable period before birth.

Expansion of the lung is very uneven at first. However, pulmonary surfactant, which is formed relatively late in fetal life, is available to stabilize open alveoli, and the lung liquid is removed by the lymphatics and capillaries. Within a short time, the functional residual capacity has almost reached its normal value, and an adequate gas-exchanging surface has been established. However, it is several days before uniform ventilation is achieved.

Circulatory Changes

A dramatic fall in pulmonary vascular resistance follows the first few breaths. In the fetus, the pulmonary arteries are exposed to the full systemic blood pressure via the DA, and their walls are very muscular. As a result, the resistance of the pulmonary circulation is exquisitely sensitive to such vasoconstrictor agents as hypoxemia, acidosis, and serotonin and to such vasodilators as acetylcholine. Several factors account for the fall in pulmonary vascular resistance at birth, including the abrupt rise in alveolar Po_2 that abolishes the hypoxic vasoconstriction and the increased volume of the lung that widens the caliber of the extra-alveolar vessels (see Figure 4-2).

Changes at or Shortly After Birth

- Baby makes strong inspiratory efforts and takes its first breath
- Large fall in pulmonary vascular resistance
- Ductus arteriosus closes, as does the foramen ovale
- Lung liquid is removed by lymphatics and capillaries

With the resulting increase in pulmonary blood flow, left atrial pressure rises and the flap-like FO quickly closes. A rise in aortic pressure resulting from the loss of the parallel umbilical circulation also increases left atrial pressure. In addition, right atrial pressure falls as the umbilical flow ceases. The DA begins to constrict a few minutes later in response to the direct action of the increased Po_2 on its smooth muscle. In addition, this constriction is aided by reductions in the levels of local and circulating prostaglandins. Flow through the DA soon reverses as the resistance of the pulmonary circulation falls.

KEY CONCEPTS

1. Exercise greatly increases O_2 uptake and CO_2 output. O_2 consumption increases linearly with work rate up to the $\dot{V}_{O_2}$ max. There is a large rise in ventilation, but cardiac output increases less.
2. The most important feature of acclimatization to high altitude is hyperventilation, which results in very low arterial Pco_2 values at extreme altitude. Polycythemia increases the O_2 concentration of the blood but is slow to develop. Other features of acclimatization include changes in oxidative enzymes and an increased capillary concentration in some tissues.
3. Patients who breathe a high concentration of O_2 are liable to develop atelectasis if an airway is obstructed, for example, by mucus. Atelectasis can also occur with air breathing, but this is much slower.

4. Following deep diving, decompression sickness may occur as a result of the formation of N_2 bubbles in the blood. These can cause pain in joints ("bends") and also CNS effects. Prevention is by gradual ascent, and treatment is by recompression.

5. Atmospheric pollutants frequently exist as aerosols that are deposited in the lung by impaction, sedimentation, or diffusion depending on the size of the particles. They are subsequently removed from the airways by the mucociliary escalator and from the alveoli by macrophages.

6. The environment of the fetus is very hypoxic, with the Po_2 in the descending aorta being less than 25 mmHg. The transition from placental to pulmonary gas exchange results in dramatic changes in the circulation, including a striking fall in pulmonary vascular resistance and eventual closure of the DA and foramen ovale.

QUESTIONS

For each question, choose the one best answer.

1. Concerning exercise,

    A. It can increase the oxygen consumption more than tenfold compared with rest.
    B. The measured respiratory exchange ratio cannot exceed 1.0.
    C. Ventilation increases less than cardiac output.
    D. At low levels of exercise, blood lactate concentrations typically rapidly increase.
    E. The change in ventilation on exercise can be fully explained by the fall in arterial pH.

2. Concerning acclimatization to high altitude,

    A. Hyperventilation is of little value.
    B. Polycythemia occurs rapidly.
    C. There is a rightward shift of the O_2 dissociation curve at extreme altitudes.
    D. The number of capillaries per unit volume in skeletal muscle falls.
    E. Changes in oxidative enzymes occur inside muscle cells.

3. If a small airway in a lung is blocked by mucus, the lung distal to this may become atelectatic. Which of the following statements is true?

    A. Atelectasis occurs faster if the person is breathing air rather than oxygen.
    B. The sum of the gas partial pressures in mixed venous blood is less than in arterial blood during air breathing.
    C. The blood flow to the atelectatic lung will rise.
    D. The absorption of a spontaneous pneumothorax is explained by a different mechanism.
    E. The elastic properties of the lung strongly resist atelectasis.

4. If helium-oxygen mixtures rather than nitrogen-oxygen mixtures (with the same oxygen concentration) are used for very deep diving,

    A. Risk of decompression sickness is reduced.
    B. Work of breathing is increased.
    C. Airway resistance is increased.
    D. Risk of O_2 toxicity is reduced.
    E. Risk of inert gas narcosis is increased.

5. If a seated astronaut makes the transition from 1G to 0G, which of the following decreases?

   A. Blood flow to the apex of the lung
   B. Ventilation to the apex of the lung
   C. Deposition of inhaled aerosol particles
   D. Thoracic blood volume
   E. P_{CO_2} in the alveoli at the apex of the lung

6. Which of the following increases by the largest percentage at maximal exercise compared with rest?

   A. Heart rate
   B. Alveolar ventilation
   C. P_{CO_2} of mixed venous blood
   D. Cardiac output
   E. Tidal volume

7. The transition from placental to pulmonary gas exchange is accompanied by

   A. Reduced arterial P_{O_2}.
   B. Rise of pulmonary vascular resistance.
   C. Closure of the ductus arteriosus.
   D. Increased blood flow through the foramen ovale.
   E. Weak respiratory efforts.

Tests of Pulmonary Function

10

FEV

This final chapter deals with pulmonary function testing, which is an important practical application of respiratory physiology in the clinic. First, we look at the forced expiration, a very simple but nevertheless very useful test. Then there are sections on ventilation-perfusion relationships, blood gases, lung mechanics, control of ventilation, and the role of exercise. The chapter concludes by emphasizing that it is more important to understand the principles of respiratory physiology contained in Chapters 1 to 9 than to concentrate on the details of pulmonary function tests.

*This chapter is only a brief introduction to pulmonary function tests. A more detailed description can be found in JB West, *Pulmonary Pathophysiology: The Essentials*, 7th ed. (Baltimore, MD: Lippincott Williams & Wilkins, 2007).

An important practical application of respiratory physiology is the testing of pulmonary function. These tests are useful in a variety of settings. The most important is the hospital pulmonary function laboratory or, on a small scale, the physician's office, where these tests help in the diagnosis and the management of patients with pulmonary or cardiac diseases. In addition, they may be valuable in deciding whether a patient is fit enough for surgery. Another use is the evaluation of disability for the purposes of insurance and workers' compensation. Again, some of the simpler tests are employed in epidemiological surveys to assess industrial hazards or to document the prevalence of disease in the community.

The role of pulmonary function tests should be kept in perspective. They are rarely a key factor in making a definitive diagnosis in a patient with lung disease. Rather, the various patterns of impaired function overlap disease entities. While the tests are often valuable for following the progress of a patient with chronic pulmonary disease and assessing the results of treatment, it is generally far more important for the medical student (or physician) to understand the principles of how the lung works (Chapters 1–9) than to concentrate only on lung function tests.

▶ Ventilation

Forced Expiration

The measurement of the forced expiratory volume (FEV) and forced vital capacity (FVC) was discussed in Chapter 7 (Figure 7-19).

Another useful way of looking at forced expirations is with *flow-volume curves* (see Figure 7-16). Figure 10-1 reminds us that after a relatively small amount of gas has been exhaled, flow is limited by airway compression and is determined by the elastic recoil force of the lung and the resistance of the

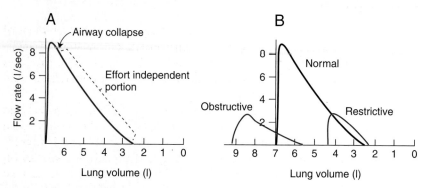

Figure 10-1. Flow-volume curves obtained by recording flow rate against volume during a forced expiration from maximum inspiration. The figures show absolute lung volumes, although these cannot be measured from single expirations. See text for details.

airways upstream of the collapse point. In *restrictive* diseases, the maximum flow rate is reduced, as is the total volume exhaled. However, if flow is related to the absolute lung volume (that is, including the residual volume, which cannot be measured from a single expiration), the flow rate is often abnormally high during the latter part of expiration because of the increased lung recoil (Figure 10-1B). By contrast, in *obstructive* diseases, the flow rate is very low in relation to lung volume, and a scooped-out appearance is often seen following the point of maximum flow.

What is the significance of these measurements of forced expirations? The FVC may be reduced at its top or bottom end (see Figure 10-1). In *restrictive* diseases, inspiration is limited by the reduced compliance of the lung or chest wall, or weakness of the inspiration muscles. In *obstructive* disease, the total lung capacity is typically abnormally large, but expiration ends prematurely. The reason for this is early airway closure brought about by increased smooth muscle tone of the bronchi, as in asthma, or loss of radial traction from surrounding parenchyma, as in emphysema. Other causes include edema of the bronchial walls, or secretions within the airways.

The $FEV_{1.0}$ (or $FEF_{25-75\%}$) is reduced by an increase in airway resistance or a reduction in elastic recoil of the lung. It is remarkably independent of expiratory effort. The reason for this is the dynamic compression of airways, which was discussed earlier (see Figure 7-18). This mechanism explains why the flow rate is independent of the resistance of the airways downstream of the collapse point but is determined by the elastic recoil pressure of the lung and the resistance of the airways upstream of the collapse point. The location of the collapse point is in the large airways, at least initially. Thus, both the increase in airway resistance and the reduction of lung elastic recoil pressure can be important factors in the reduction of the $FEV_{1.0}$, as, for example, in pulmonary emphysema.

Lung Volumes

The determination of lung volumes by spirometry and the measurement of functional residual capacity (FRC) by helium dilution and body plethysmography were discussed earlier (see Figures 2-2 through 2-4). The FRC can also be found by having the subject breathe 100% O_2 for several minutes and washing all the N_2 out of the subject's lung.

Suppose that the lung volume is V_1 and that the total volume of gas exhaled over 7 minutes is V_2 and that its concentration of N_2 is C_2. We know that the concentration of N_2 in the lung before washout was 80%, and we can measure the concentration left in the lung by sampling end-expired gas with an N_2 meter at the lips. Call this concentration C_3. Then, assuming no net change in the amount of N_2, we can write $V_1 \times 380 = (V_1 \times C_3) + (V_2 \times C_2)$. Thus, V_1 can be derived. A disadvantage of this method is that the concentration of nitrogen in the gas collected over 7 minutes is very low, and a small error in its measurement leads to a larger error in calculated lung volume. In addition, some of the N_2 that is washed out comes from body tissues, and this should be allowed for. This method, like the helium dilution technique, measures only ventilated lung volume, whereas, as we saw in the discussion of Figure 2-4, the body plethysmograph method includes gas trapped behind closed airways.

The measurement of anatomic dead space by Fowler's method was described earlier (see Figure 2-6).

▶ Diffusion

The principles of the measurement of the diffusing capacity for carbon monoxide by the single-breath method were discussed on p. 32. The diffusing capacity for O_2 is very difficult to measure, and it is only done as a research procedure.

▶ Blood Flow

The measurement of total pulmonary blood flow by the Fick principle and by the indicator dilution method was discussed on p. 45.

▶ Ventilation-Perfusion Relationships

Topographical Distribution of Ventilation and Perfusion

Regional differences of ventilation and blood flow can be measured using radioactive xenon, as briefly described earlier (see Figures 2-7 and 4-7).

Inequality of Ventilation

This can be measured by single-breath and multiple-breath methods. The *single-breath method* is very similar to that described by Fowler for measuring anatomic dead space (Figure 2-6). There we saw that if the N_2 concentration at the lips is measured following a single breath of O_2, the N_2 concentration of the expired alveolar gas is almost uniform, giving a nearly flat "alveolar plateau." This reflects the approximately uniform dilution of the alveolar gas by the inspired O_2. By contrast, in patients with lung disease, the alveolar N_2 concentration continues to rise during expiration. This is caused by the uneven dilution of the alveolar N_2 by inspired O_2.

The reason the concentration rises is that the poorly ventilated alveoli (those in which the N_2 has been diluted least) always empty last, presumably because they have long time constants (see Figures 7-20 and 10-4). In practice, the change in N_2 percentage concentration between 750 and 1250 ml

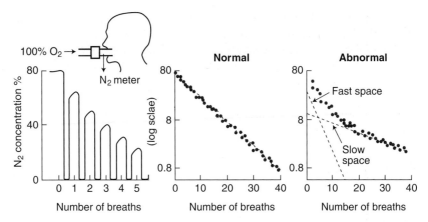

Figure 10-2. N_2 washout obtained when a subject breathes 100% O_2. Normal lungs give an almost linear plot of N_2 concentration against number of breaths on semilogarithmic paper, but this plot is nonlinear when uneven ventilation is present.

of expired volume is often used as an index of uneven ventilation. This is a simple, quick, and useful test.

The *multiple-breath method* is based on the rate of washout of N_2, as shown in Figure 10-2. The subject is connected to a source of 100% O_2, and a fast-responding N_2 meter samples gas at the lips. If the ventilation of the lung were uniform, the N_2 concentration would be reduced by the same *fraction* with each breath. For example, if the tidal volume (excluding dead space) were equal to the FRC, the N_2 concentration would halve with each breath. In general, the N_2 concentration is $FRC/[FRC + (V_T - V_D)]$ times that of the previous breath, where V_T and V_D are the tidal volume and anatomic dead space, respectively. Because the N_2 is reduced by the same fraction with each breath, the plot of log N_2 concentration against breath number would be a straight line (see Figure 10-2) if the lung behaved as a single, uniformly ventilated compartment. This is very nearly the case in normal subjects.

In patients with lung disease, however, the nonuniform ventilation results in a curved plot because different lung units have their N_2 diluted at different rates. Thus, fast-ventilated alveoli cause a rapid initial fall in N_2, whereas slow-ventilated spaces are responsible for the long tail of the washout (see Figure 10-2).

Inequality of Ventilation-Perfusion Ratios

One way of assessing the mismatch of ventilation and blood flow within the diseased lung is that introduced by Riley. This is based on measurements of P_{O_2} and P_{CO_2} in arterial blood and expired gas (the principles were briefly described in Chapter 5). In practice, expired gas and arterial blood are

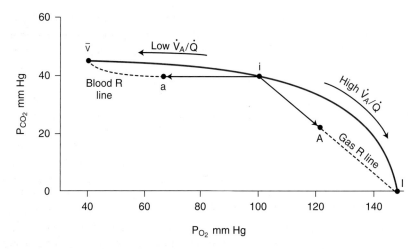

Figure 10-3. O_2-CO_2 diagram showing the ideal point (i), that is, the hypothetical composition of alveolar gas and end-capillary blood when no ventilation-perfusion inequality is present. As inequality develops, the arterial (a) and alveolar (A) points diverge along their respective R (respiratory exchange ratio) lines. The mixed alveolar-arterial PO_2 difference is the horizontal distance between the points.

collected simultaneously from the patient, and various indices of ventilation-perfusion inequality are computed.

One useful measurement is the *alveolar-arterial* Po_2 difference. We saw in Figure 5-11 how this develops because of regional differences of gas exchange in the normal lung. Figure 10-3 is an O_2-CO_2 diagram that allows us to examine this development more closely. First, suppose that there is no ventilation-perfusion inequality and that all the lung units are represented by a single point (i) on the ventilation-perfusion line. This is known as the "ideal" point. Now as ventilation-perfusion inequality develops, the lung units begin to spread away from i toward both $\bar{v}$ (low ventilation-perfusion ratios) and I (high ventilation-perfusion ratios) (compare Figure 5-7). When this happens, the mixed capillary blood (a) and mixed alveolar gas (A) also diverge from i. They do so along lines i to $\bar{v}$ and i to I, which represent a constant respiratory exchange ratio (CO_2 output/O_2 uptake), because this is determined by the metabolism of the body tissues.[†]

The horizontal distance between A and a represents the (*mixed*) *alveolar-arterial O_2* difference. In practice, this can only be measured easily if ventilation is essentially uniform but blood flow is uneven, because only then can a representative sample of mixed alveolar gas be obtained. This is sometimes the case in pulmonary embolism. More frequently, the Po_2 difference between ideal

---

[†]In this necessarily simplified description, some details are omitted. For example, the mixed venous point alters when ventilation-perfusion inequality develops.

alveolar gas and arterial blood is calculated—the (*ideal*) *alveolar-arterial O$_2$* difference. The ideal alveolar Po$_2$ can be calculated from the alveolar gas equation that relates the Po$_2$ of any lung unit to the composition of the inspired gas, the respiratory exchange ratio, and the Pco$_2$ of the unit. In the case of ideal alveoli, the Pco$_2$ is taken to be the same as arterial blood because the line along which point i moves is so nearly horizontal. Note that this alveolar-arterial Po$_2$ difference is caused by units between i and $\bar{v}$, that is, those with low ventilation-perfusion ratios.

Two more indices of ventilation-perfusion inequality are frequently derived. One is *physiologic shunt* (also called *venous admixture*). For this, we pretend that all of the leftward movement of the arterial point (a) away from the ideal point (i) (that is, the hypoxemia) is caused by the addition of mixed venous blood ($\bar{v}$) to ideal blood (i). This is not so fanciful as it first seems, because units with very low ventilation-perfusion ratios put out blood that has essentially the same composition as mixed venous blood (see Figures 5-6 and 5-7). In practice, the shunt equation (see Figure 5-3) is used in the following form:

$$\frac{\dot{Q}_{PS}}{\dot{Q}_T} = \frac{Ci_{O_2} - Ca_{O_2}}{Ci_{O_2} - C\bar{v}_{O_2}}$$

where $\dot{Q}_{PS}/\dot{Q}_T$ refers to the ratio of the physiologic shunt to total flow. The O$_2$ concentration of ideal blood is calculated from the ideal Po$_2$ and O$_2$ dissociation curve.

The other index is *alveolar dead space*. Here we pretend that all of the movement of the alveolar point (A) away from the ideal point (i) is caused by the addition of inspired gas (I) to ideal gas. Again, this is not such an outrageous notion as it may first appear because units with very high ventilation-perfusion ratios behave very much like point I. After all, a unit with an infinitely high ventilation-perfusion ratio contains gas that has the same composition as inspired air (see Figures 5-6 and 5-7). The Bohr equation for dead space (see p. 22) is used in the following form:

$$\frac{VD_{alv}}{VT} = \frac{Pi_{CO_2} - PA_{CO_2}}{Pi_{CO_2}}$$

where A refers to expired alveolar gas. The result is called *alveolar dead space* to distinguish it from the *anatomic dead space*, that is, the volume of the conducting airways. Because expired alveolar gas is often difficult to collect without contamination by the anatomic dead space, the mixed expired CO$_2$ is often measured. The result is called the *physiologic dead space*, which includes components from the alveolar dead space and anatomic dead space. Because

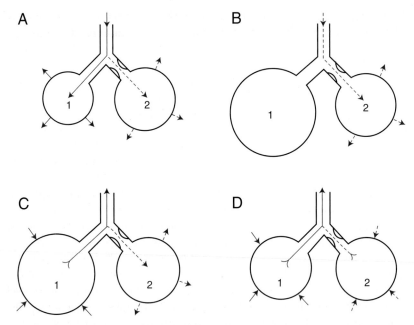

Figure 10-4. Effects of uneven time constants on ventilation. Compartment 2 has a partially obstructed airway and, therefore, a long time constant (compare Figure 7-20). During inspiration **(A)**, gas is slow to enter it, and it therefore continues to fill after the rest of the lung (1) has stopped moving **(B)**. Indeed, at the beginning of the expiration **(C)**, the abnormal region (2) may still be inhaling while the rest of the lung has begun to exhale. In **D**, both regions are exhaling, but compartment 2 lags behind compartment 1. At higher frequencies, the tidal volume to the abnormal region becomes progressively smaller.

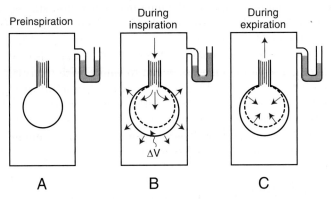

Figure 10-5. Measurement of airway resistance with the body plethysmograph. During inspiration, the alveolar gas is expanded, and box pressure therefore rises. From this, alveolar pressure can be calculated. The difference between alveolar and mouth pressure, divided by flow, gives airway resistance (see text).

Before inspiration (A), the box pressure is atmospheric. At the onset of inspiration, the pressure in the alveoli falls as the alveolar gas expands by a volume ΔV. This compresses the gas in the box, and from its change in pressure ΔV can be calculated (compare Figure 2-4). If lung volume is known, ΔV can be converted into alveolar pressure using Boyle's law. Flow is measured simultaneously, and thus airway resistance is obtained. The measurement is made during expiration in the same way. Lung volume is determined as described in Figure 2-4.

Airway resistance can also be measured during normal breathing from an intrapleural pressure record as obtained with an esophageal balloon (see Figure 7-13). However, in this case, tissue viscous resistance is included as well (see p. 125). Intrapleural pressure reflects two sets of forces, those opposing the elastic recoil of the lung and those overcoming resistance to air and tissue flow. It is possible to subtract the pressure caused by the recoil forces during quiet breathing because this is proportional to lung volume (if compliance is constant). The subtraction is done with an electrical circuit. We are then left with a plot of pressure against flow that gives (airway + tissue) resistance. This method is not satisfactory in lungs with severe airway disease because the uneven time constants prevent all regions from moving together (see Figure 10-4).

Closing Volume

Early disease in small airways can be sought by using the single-breath N_2 washout (see Figure 2-6) and thus exploiting the topographical differences of ventilation (see Figures 7-8 and 7-9). Suppose a subject takes a vital capacity breath of 100% O_2, and during the subsequent exhalation the N_2 concentration at the lips is measured (Figure 10-6). Four phases can be recognized.

First, pure dead space is exhaled (1), followed by a mixture of dead space and alveolar gas (2), and then pure alveolar gas (3). Toward the end of expiration, an abrupt increase in N_2 concentration is seen (4). This signals closure of airways at the base of the lung (see Figure 7-9) and is caused by preferential emptying of the apex, which has a relatively high concentration of N_2. The reason for the higher N_2 at the apex is that during a vital capacity breath of O_2, this region expands less (see Figure 7-9), and, therefore, the N_2 there is less diluted with O_2. Thus, the volume of the lung at which dependent airways begin to close can be read off the tracing.

In young normal subjects, the closing volume is about 10% of the vital capacity (VC). It increases steadily with age and is equal to about 40% of the VC, that is, the FRC, at about the age of 65 years. Relatively small amounts of disease in the small airways apparently increase the closing volume. Sometimes the *closing capacity* is reported. This is the closing volume plus the residual volume.

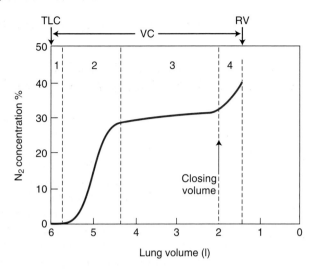

Figure 10-6. Measurement of the closing volume. If a vital capacity inspiration of 100% O_2 is followed by a full expiration, four phases in the N_2 concentration measured at the lips can be recognized (see text). The last is caused by preferential emptying of the upper part of the lung after the lower-zone airways have closed.

▶ Control of Ventilation

The responsiveness of the chemoreceptors and respiratory center to CO_2 can be measured by having the subject rebreathe into a rubber bag, as discussed on p. 139. We saw that the alveolar Po_2 also affects ventilation, so that if the response to CO_2 alone is required, the inspired Po_2 should be kept above 200 mm Hg to avoid any hypoxic drive. The ventilatory response to hypoxia can be measured in a similar way if the subject rebreathes from a bag with a low Po_2 but constant Pco_2.

▶ Exercise

Additional information about pulmonary function can often be obtained if tests are made when the subject exercises. As discussed at the beginning of Chapter 9, the resting lung has enormous reserves; its ventilation, blood flow, O_2 and CO_2 transfer, and diffusing capacity can be increased severalfold on exercise. Frequently, patients with early disease have pulmonary function tests that are within normal limits at rest, but abnormalities are revealed when the respiratory system is stressed by exercise.

Methods of providing controlled exercise include the treadmill and bicycle ergometer. Measurements most often made on exercise include total ventilation, pulse rate, O_2 uptake, CO_2 output, respiratory exchange ratio, arterial blood gases, and the diffusing capacity of the lung for carbon monoxide.

▶ Perspective on Tests of Pulmonary Function

In this chapter, we have touched on some of the lung function tests that are presently available. In conclusion, it should be emphasized that not all these tests are commonly used in a hospital pulmonary function laboratory. Only a few can be used in a doctor's office or on an epidemiological survey.

The most useful and simplest test in the clinical setting is the *forced expiration*. It does not matter much which indices are derived from this test, but the $FEV_{1.0}$ and FVC are very frequently reported. Next, the ability to measure *arterial blood gases* is essential if patients with respiratory failure are being managed, and is often valuable in any case. After these, the relative importance of tests becomes more a matter of personal preference, but a well-equipped pulmonary function laboratory would be able to measure lung volumes, inequality of ventilation, alveolar-arterial Po_2 difference, physiologic dead space and shunt, diffusing capacity for carbon monoxide, airway resistance, lung compliance, ventilatory response to CO_2 and hypoxia, and the patient's response to exercise. In large laboratories, more specialized measurements such as the topographical distribution of ventilation and blood flow would be available.

KEY CONCEPTS

1. The measurement of a single forced expiration is simple to perform and often very informative. Specific patterns occur in obstructive and restrictive lung disease.
2. Arterial blood gases can be quickly measured with blood-gas electrodes, and this information is often essential in the management of critically ill patients.
3. The degree of ventilation-perfusion inequality in a diseased lung can be assessed from an arterial blood sample by calculating the alveolar-arterial Po_2 difference.
4. Lung volumes and airway resistance can be measured in a body plethysmograph relatively easily.
5. Exercise testing can be valuable in detecting small amounts of lung disease.

QUESTIONS

For each question, choose the one best answer.

1. Concerning the 1-second forced expiratory volume,

   A. The test can be used to assess the efficacy of bronchodilators.
   B. It is unaffected by dynamic compression of the airways.
   C. It is reduced in patients with pulmonary fibrosis but not chronic obstructive pulmonary disease.
   D. It is normal in patients with asthma.
   E. The test is difficult to perform.

2. The following may reduce the FEV$_1$ in a patient with chronic obstructive pulmonary disease:

   A. Hypertrophy of the diaphragm.
   B. Administration of a bronchodilator drug.
   C. Increased expiratory effort.
   D. Loss of radial traction on the airways.
   E. Increased elastic recoil of the lung.

3. Concerning the single-breath nitrogen test for uneven ventilation,

   A. The slope of the alveolar plateau is reduced in chronic bronchitis compared with normal.
   B. The slope occurs because well-ventilated units empty later in expiration than poorly ventilated units.
   C. The last exhaled gas comes from the base of the lung.
   D. A similar procedure can be used to measure the anatomic dead space.
   E. The test is very time consuming.

4. In the assessment of ventilation-perfusion inequality based on measurements of Po$_2$ and Pco$_2$ in arterial blood and expired gas,

   A. The ideal alveolar Po$_2$ is calculated using the expired Pco$_2$.
   B. The alveolar Po$_2$ is calculated from the alveolar gas equation.
   C. $\dot{V}_A / \dot{Q}$ inequality reduces the alveolar-arterial Po$_2$ difference.
   D. $\dot{V}_A / \dot{Q}$ inequality reduces the physiologic shunt.
   E. $\dot{V}_A / \dot{Q}$ inequality reduces the physiologic dead space.

5. If a seated normal subject exhales to residual volume (RV),

   A. The volume of gas remaining in the lung is more than half of the vital capacity.
   B. The Pco$_2$ of the expired gas falls just before the end of expiration.
   C. If the mouthpiece is closed at RV and the subject completely relaxes, the pressure in the airways is greater than atmospheric pressure.
   D. Intrapleural pressure exceeds alveolar pressure at RV.
   E. All small airways in the lung are closed at RV.

Symbols, Units, and Equations

▶ SYMBOLS

Primary Symbols

C   Concentration of gas in blood
F   Fractional concentration in dry gas
P   Pressure or partial pressure
Q   Volume of blood
$\dot{Q}$ Volume of blood per unit time
R   Respiratory exchange ratio
S   Saturation of hemoglobin with O_2
V   Volume of gas
$\dot{V}$ Volume of gas per unit time

Secondary Symbols for Gas Phase

A   Alveolar
B   Barometric
D   Dead space
E   Expired
I   Inspired
L   Lung
T   Tidal

Secondary Symbols for Blood Phase

a   arterial
c   capillary
c′   end-capillary
i   ideal
v   venous
$\bar{v}$ mixed venous

Examples

O_2 concentration in arterial blood, Ca_{O_2}
Fractional concentration of N_2 in expired gas, $F_{E_{N_2}}$
Partial pressure of O_2 in mixed venous blood, $P\bar{v}_{O_2}$

▶ UNITS

Traditional metric units have been used in this book. Pressures are given in mm Hg; the torr is an almost identical unit.

In Europe, SI (Système International) units are commonly used. Most of these are familiar, but the kilopascal, the unit of pressure, is confusing at first. One kilopascal = 7.5 mm Hg (approximately).

▶ EQUATIONS

Gas Laws

General gas law : $PV = RT$

where T is temperature and R is a constant. This equation is used to correct gas volumes for changes of water vapor pressure and temperature. For example, ventilation is conventionally reported at BTPS, that is, body temperature (37°C), ambient pressure, and saturated with water vapor, because it then corresponds to the volume changes of the lung. By contrast, gas volumes in blood are expressed as STPD, that is, standard temperature (0°C or 273 K) and pressure (760 mm Hg) and dry, as is usual in chemistry. To convert a gas volume at BTPS to one at STPD, multiply by

$$\frac{273}{310} \times \frac{P_B - 47}{760}$$

where 47 mm Hg is the water vapor pressure at 37°C.

Boyle's law $P_1 V_1 = P_2 V_2$ (temperature constant)

and

Charles' law $\dfrac{V_1}{V_2} = \dfrac{T_1}{T_2}$ (pressure constant)

are special cases of the general gas law.

Avogadro's law states that equal volumes of different gases at the same temperature and pressure contain the same number of molecules. A gram molecule, for example, 32 g of O_2, occupies 22.4 liters at STPD.

Dalton's law states that the partial pressure of a gas (x) in a gas mixture is the pressure that this gas would exert if it occupied the total volume of the mixture in the absence of the other components.

Thus, $P_x = P \cdot F_x$, where P is the total dry gas pressure, since F_x refers to dry gas. In gas with a water vapor pressure of 47 mm Hg,

$$P_x = (P_B - 47) \cdot F_x$$

Also, in the alveoli, $P_{O_2} + P_{CO_2} + P_{N_2} + P_{H_2O} = P_B$.

The *partial pressure of a gas in solution* is its partial pressure in a gas mixture that is in equilibrium with the solution.

Henry's law states that the concentration of gas dissolved in a liquid is proportional to its partial pressure. Thus, $C_x = K \cdot P_x$.

Ventilation

$$V_T = V_D + V_A$$

where V_A here refers to the volume of alveolar gas in the tidal volume

$$\dot{V}_A = \dot{V}_E - \dot{V}_D$$

$$\dot{V}_{CO_2} = \dot{V}_A \cdot F_{A_{CO_2}} \quad (\text{both } \dot{V} \text{ measured at BTPS})$$

$$\dot{V}_A = \frac{\dot{V}_{CO_2}}{P_{A_{CO_2}}} \times K \ (\text{alveolar ventilation equation})$$

If $\dot{V}_A$ is BTPS and $\dot{V}_{CO_2}$ is STPD, K = 0.863. In normal subjects, Pa_{CO_2} is nearly equal to $P_{A_{CO_2}}$.

Bohr equation

$$\frac{V_D}{V_T} = \frac{P_{A_{CO_2}} - P_{E_{CO_2}}}{P_{A_{CO_2}}}$$

Or, using arterial P_{CO_2},

$$\frac{V_D}{V_T} = \frac{Pa_{CO_2} - P_{E_{CO_2}}}{Pa_{CO_2}}$$

This gives *physiologic dead space*.

Diffusion

In the *gas phase*, *Graham's law* states that the rate of diffusion of a gas is inversely proportional to the square root of its molecular weight.

In *liquid* or a *tissue slice*, *Fick's law** states that the volume of gas per unit time that diffuses across a tissue sheet is given by

$$\dot{V}_{gas} = \frac{A}{T} \cdot D \cdot (P_1 - P_2)$$

where A and T are the area and thickness of the sheet, P_1 and P_2 are the partial pressure of the gas on the two sides, and D is a diffusion constant sometimes called the permeability coefficient of the tissue for that gas.

This *diffusion constant* is related to the solubility (Sol) and the molecular weight (MW) of the gas:

$$D \alpha \frac{Sol}{\sqrt{MW}}$$

When the diffusing capacity of the lung (D_L) is measured with carbon monoxide and the capillary P_{CO} is taken as zero,

$$D_L = \frac{\dot{V}_{CO}}{P_{A_{CO}}}$$

D_L is made up of two components. One is the diffusing capacity of the alveolar membrane (D_M), and the other depends on the volume of capillary blood (V_c) and the rate of reaction of CO with hemoglobin, θ:

$$\frac{1}{D_L} = \frac{1}{D_M} + \frac{1}{\theta \cdot V_c}$$

Blood Flow

Fick principle

$$\dot{Q} = \frac{\dot{V}_{O_2}}{Ca_{O_2} - C\bar{v}_{O_2}}$$

---

*Fick's law was originally expressed in terms of concentrations, but partial pressures are more convenient for us.

Pulmonary vascular resistance

$$PVR = \frac{P_{art} - P_{ven}}{\dot{Q}}$$

where P_{art} and P_{ven} are the mean pulmonary arterial and venous pressures, respectively.

Starling's law of fluid exchange across the capillaries

$$\text{Net flow out} = K[(P_c - P_i) - \sigma(\pi_c - \pi_i)]$$

where i refers to the interstitial fluid around the capillary, π refers to the colloid osmotic pressure, σ is the reflection coefficient, and K is the filtration coefficient.

Ventilation-Perfusion Relationships

Alveolar gas equation

$$P_{A_{O_2}} = P_{I_{O_2}} - \frac{P_{A_{CO_2}}}{R} + \left[P_{A_{CO_2}} \cdot F_{I_{O_2}} \cdot \frac{1-R}{R} \right]$$

This is only valid if there is no CO_2 in inspired gas. The term in square brackets is a relatively small correction factor when air is breathed (2 mm Hg when $P_{CO_2} = 40$, $F_{I_{O_2}} = 0.21$, and R = 0.8). Thus, a useful approximation is

$$P_{A_{O_2}} = P_{I_{O_2}} - \frac{P_{A_{CO_2}}}{R}$$

Respiratory exchange ratio
If no CO_2 is present in the inspired gas,

$$R = \frac{\dot{V}_{CO_2}}{\dot{V}_{O_2}} = \frac{P_{E_{CO_2}}(1 - F_{I_{O_2}})}{P_{I_{O_2}} - P_{E_{O_2}} - (P_{E_{CO_2}} \cdot F_{I_{O_2}})}$$

Venous to arterial shunt

$$\frac{\dot{Q}_S}{\dot{Q}_T} = \frac{Cc'_{O_2} - Ca_{O_2}}{Cc'_{O_2} - C\bar{v}_{O_2}}$$

where c′ means end-capillary.

Ventilation-perfusion ratio equation

$$\frac{\dot{V}_A}{\dot{Q}} = \frac{8.63R(Ca_{O_2} - C\bar{v}_{O_2})}{P_{A_{CO_2}}}$$

where blood gas concentrations are in ml·100 ml⁻¹.

Physiologic shunt

$$\frac{\dot{Q}_{PS}}{\dot{Q}_T} = \frac{Ci_{O_2} - Ca_{O_2}}{Ci_{O_2} - C\bar{v}_{O_2}}$$

Alveolar dead space

$$\frac{V_D}{V_T} = \frac{Pi_{CO_2} - P_{A_{CO_2}}}{Pi_{CO_2}}$$

The equation for *physiologic dead space* is on p. 181.

Blood Gases and pH

O_2 dissolved in blood

$$C_{O_2} = Sol \cdot P_{O_2}$$

where Sol is 0.003 ml O_2·100 ml blood⁻¹·mm Hg⁻¹.

Henderson-Hasselbalch equation

$$pH = pK_A + \log\frac{(HCO_3^-)}{(CO_2)}$$

The pK_A for this system is normally 6.1. If HCO_3^- and CO_2 concentrations are in millimoles per liter, CO_2 can be replaced by Pco_2 (mm Hg) × 0.030.

Mechanics of Breathing

Compliance = $\Delta V/\Delta P$

Specific compliance = $\Delta V/(V \cdot \Delta P)$

Laplace equation for pressure caused by surface tension of a sphere

$$P = \frac{2T}{r}$$

where r is the radius and T is the surface tension. Note that for a soap bubble, P = 4T/r, because there are two surfaces.

Poiseuille's law for laminar flow

$$\dot{V} = \frac{P\pi r^4}{8nl}$$

where n is the coefficient of viscosity[†] and P is the pressure difference across the length l.

Reynolds number

$$Re = \frac{2rvd}{n}$$

where v is average linear velocity of the gas, d is its density, and n is its viscosity. *Pressure drop* for laminar flow, $P\alpha\dot{V}$, but for turbulent flow, $P\alpha\dot{V}_2$ (approximately).

Airway resistance

$$\frac{P_{alv} - P_{mouth}}{\dot{V}}$$

where P_{alv} and P_{mouth} refer to alveolar and mouth pressures, respectively.

[†]This is a corruption of the Greek letter η for those of us who have little Latin and less Greek.

Answers

Chapter 1

1. D is correct. The capillary walls are so thin that if the pressure in them rises too much, they are damaged and leak plasma or blood, a condition known as stress failure. The other choices are incorrect because the thinnest part of the blood-gas barrier is about 0.3 μm thick, its total area exceeds 50 square meters, almost all of the area of the alveolar wall is occupied by capillaries, and oxygen crosses the barrier by passive diffusion.

2. B is correct. See the caption to Figure 1-1.

3. B is correct. The calculation is $0.2093 \times (247 - 47)$.

4. E is correct. The combined cross sectional area of the alveolar ducts is so great (Figure 1-5) that gas diffusion is the main mode of transport rather than convection. The other choices are incorrect. The volume of the conducting airways is about 150 ml, the volume of the lung at FRC is about 3 liters, a respiratory bronchiole but not a terminal bronchiole has alveoli in its walls, and there are about 16 branches of the conducting airways before the first alveoli appear.

5. D is correct (see Figure 3-2). The other choices are incorrect because the branching pattern of the arteries, not the veins, matches the airways, the average diameter of the capillaries is about 7 to 10 μm, the flow in the bronchial circulation is very small compared to the pulmonary circulation, and the mean pressure in the pulmonary artery is about 15 mm Hg.

Chapter 2

1. B is correct. The FRC includes the residual volume and cannot be measured with a simple spirometer. All the other choices can be measured with a spirometer and stopwatch (see Figure 2-2).

2. D is correct. An acinus is that portion of the lung supplied by a terminal bronchiole. The other choices are incorrect because all the oxygen uptake occurs in the acini, the change in volume of the acini during breathing is greater than that of the whole lung because the volume of the conducting airways remains almost constant, the volume of the acini is about 95% of the total volume of the lung at FRC (FRC is about 3 liters, conducting airways are about 150 ml), and the ventilation of the

acini is greater at the base than the apex of the upright lung at FRC (see Figure 7-8).

3. C is correct. If the volume of the FRC is denoted as V, the amount of helium initially in the spirometer is 5×0.1, and the amount after dilution is $(5 + V) \times 0.06$. Therefore, $V = 0.5/0.06 - 5$ or 3.3 liters.

4. D is correct. When the patient makes an expiratory effort, he compresses the gas in the lung so that airway pressure increases and lung volume decreases slightly. The reduction of volume in the lung means that the box gas volume increases and therefore, its pressure decreases according to Boyle's law.

5. B is correct. The alveolar ventilation equation states that if CO_2 production is constant, the alveolar P_{CO_2} is inversely related to the alveolar ventilation. Therefore, if the ventilation is increased 3 times, the P_{CO_2} will be reduced to a third of its former value, that is, 33%.

6. B is correct. The equation states that the ratio equals $(P_A - P_E)/P_A$, or $(40 - 30)/40$, that is 0.25.

Chapter 3

1. C is correct. The law states that the diffusion rate is proportional to the solubility but inversely proportional to the square root of the density. Therefore, the ratio of X to Y is $4/(\sqrt{4})$ or $4/2$, that is, 2.

2. E is correct. The equation is CO uptake divided by alveolar P_{CO}, or 30/0.5, that is, 60 ml·min^{-1}·mm Hg^{-1}

3. E is correct. The question is really asking for the conditions under which oxygen uptake or CO_2 output are diffusion limited. The only correct answer is maximal oxygen uptake at extreme altitude (see Figure 3-3B). None of the other choices refer to situations where gas transfer is diffusion limited. The only possible alternative choice is B, but resting oxygen uptake is unlikely to be diffusion limited when a subject breathes 10% oxygen. Furthermore, in all these questions, we are looking for the one best answer, and this is clearly E.

4. C is correct. This question is testing the concepts of diffusion and perfusion limitation. Carbon monoxide is a diffusion-limited gas, so it is transferred into the blood along the whole length of the capillary, and there is a large difference in partial pressure between alveolar gas and end-capillary blood (Figure 3-2). The opposite is true for nitrous oxide.

5. C is correct. Breathing oxygen reduces the measured diffusing capacity for carbon monoxide because the oxygen competes with carbon monoxide for hemoglobin, and therefore, the rate of reaction of carbon monoxide with hemoglobin (θ) is reduced. The other choices are incorrect because the reason for using carbon monoxide to measure the diffusing capacity of the

lung is because it is a diffusion-limited gas, not because it diffuses slowly across the blood-gas barrier (its diffusion rate is not very different from that of oxygen). Diffusion limitation of oxygen transfer during exercise is more likely to occur at high altitude than sea level, and the diffusing capacity is increased by exercise and decreased by pulmonary fibrosis.

6. D is correct. Exercise increases the diffusing capacity because of recruitment and distension of pulmonary capillaries. Emphysema, asbestosis, pulmonary embolism, and severe anemia reduce the diffusing capacity because of a reduction in surface area of the blood-gas barrier, an increase in its thickness, or a reduction of the volume of blood in the pulmonary capillaries.

Chapter 4

1. D is correct. The flows in the systemic and pulmonary circulations are the same, but the mean pressure difference across the pulmonary circulation is about $(15 - 5)$ mm Hg whereas that for the systemic circulation is about $(100 - 2)$ mm Hg (see Figure 4-1). Therefore, the ratio is about 10:1.

2. B is correct (Figure 4-3). The other choices are incorrect because the tension in the surrounding alveolar walls tends to pull the extra-alveolar vessels open, these vessels are not exposed to alveolar pressure, hypoxic pulmonary vasoconstriction occurs mainly in the small arteries, and the caliber of the extra-alveolar vessels is increased by lung inflation (see Figures 4-2 and 4-6).

3. E is correct. The pulmonary vascular resistance is given by the pressure difference divided by the flow, or $(55 - 5)$ divided by 3, that is, approximately 17 mm Hg·liter^{-1}·min.

4. D is correct. Distension of pulmonary capillaries lowers their vascular resistance. However, a decrease in both pulmonary arterial and pulmonary venous pressure reduces capillary pressure (other things remaining equal), and resistance therefore rises. The same is true of an increase in alveolar pressure, which tends to compress the capillaries. Alveolar hypoxia increases vascular resistance because of hypoxic pulmonary vasoconstriction.

5. C is correct. The Fick principle states that the cardiac output is equal to the oxygen consumption divided by the arterial-venous oxygen concentration difference. The latter is $(20 - 16)$ ml·100 ml^{-1} or $(200 - 160)$ ml·liter^{-1}. Therefore, the cardiac output is equal to $300/(200 - 160)$ or 7.5 liters·min^{-1}.

6. D is correct. In zone 2, flow is determined by arterial minus alveolar pressure. The other choices are incorrect because arterial pressure exceeds alveolar pressure, alveolar pressure exceeds venous pressure, and of course arterial pressure exceeds venous pressure.

7. D is correct. Acutely increasing pulmonary venous pressure will raise capillary pressure and result in recruitment and distension of the capillaries. The

other choices are incorrect because removing one lung greatly reduces the vascular bed, 10% oxygen breathing results in hypoxic pulmonary vasoconstriction, reducing lung volume to residual volume increases the resistance of the extra-alveolar vessels, and mechanically ventilating the lung with positive pressure increases the alveolar pressure and therefore tends to compress the capillaries.

8. B is correct. The great reduction in pulmonary vascular resistance during the transition from placental to air respiration is largely brought about by the release of hypoxic pulmonary vasoconstriction. The other choices are incorrect because the P_{O_2} of alveolar gas is much more important than the P_{O_2} of mixed venous blood, CO_2 uptake is irrelevant, the constriction partly diverts blood flow from poorly ventilated, not well-ventilated regions of diseased lungs, and the inhalation of nitric oxide partly reverses hypoxic pulmonary vasoconstriction.

9. A is correct. The movement of fluid between the capillary lumen and interstitium obeys Starling's Law. In the example given, the hydrostatic pressure difference moving fluid out of the capillary is $(3 - 0)$, and the colloid osmotic pressure tending to move fluid into the capillary is $(25 - 5)$ mm Hg. Therefore, the net pressure in mm Hg moving fluid into the capillaries is 17 mm Hg.

10. D is correct. Leukotrienes are almost completely removed from the blood in the pulmonary circulation (see Table 4-1). The other choices are incorrect because angiotensin I is converted to angiotensin II, bradykinin is largely inactivated, serotonin is almost completely removed, and erythropoietin is unchanged.

Chapter 5

1. D is correct. The P_{O_2} of moist inspired gas is given by $0.2093 \times (447 - 47)$, that is, about 84 mm Hg.

2. B is correct. To answer this question we first use the alveolar ventilation equation, which states that if the CO_2 output is unchanged, the P_{CO_2} is inversely proportional to the alveolar ventilation. Therefore, since alveolar ventilation was halved, the arterial P_{CO_2} was increased from 40 to 80 mm Hg. Then we use the alveolar gas equation $P_{A_{O_2}} = P_{I_{O_2}} - P_{A_{CO_2}} / R + F$, and we ignore F because it is small. Therefore, $P_{A_{O_2}} = 149 - 80/0.8$, which is approximately equal to 50 mm Hg.

3. A is correct. The last equation above shows that to return the arterial P_{O_2} to its normal value of about 100, we need to raise the inspired P_{O_2} from 149 to 199 mm Hg. Recall that the inspired P_{O_2} equals the fractional concentration of oxygen $\times (760 - 47)$. Therefore, the fractional concentration = 199/713 or 0.28 approximately. Thus, the inspired oxygen concentration as a percentage has to be increased from 21 to 28, that is, by 7%. Note that

this example emphasizes how powerful the effect of increasing the inspired oxygen concentration on the arterial P_{O_2} is when hypoxemia is caused by hypoventilation.

4. B is correct. This question is about the shunt equation shown in Figure 5-3. The shunt as a fraction of cardiac output is given by $(Cc' - Ca)/(Cc' - Cv)$. Inserting the values gives the shunt as $(20 - 18)/(20 - 14)$ or $2/6$, that is, 33%.

5. B is correct. The inspired $P_{O_2} = 0.21 \times (247 - 47)$ or 42 mm Hg. Therefore, using the alveolar gas equation as stated above and neglecting the small factor F, the alveolar P_{O_2} is given by $42 - P_{CO_2}/R$ where R is equal to or less than 1. Therefore to maintain an alveolar P_{O_2} of 34 mm Hg, the alveolar P_{CO_2} cannot exceed 8 mmHg.

6. E is correct. This question is testing knowledge about the effects of ventilation-perfusion inequality on O_2 and CO_2 transfer by the lung. VA/Q inequality impairs the transfer of both O_2 and CO_2 so that, other things being equal, this patient would have both a low arterial P_{O_2} and high P_{CO_2}. However, by increasing the ventilation to the alveoli, the P_{CO_2} can be brought back to normal, but the P_{O_2} cannot. The reason for this is the different shapes of the O_2 and CO_2 dissociation curves. The other choices are incorrect because, as already stated, VA/Q does interfere with CO_2 elimination. The statements that much of the CO_2 is carried as bicarbonate, the formation of carbonic acid is accelerated by carbonic anhydrase, and CO_2 diffuses much faster through tissue than O_2 are true but are not the explanation for the normal P_{O_2} despite the hypoxemia.

7. A is correct. The apex of the upright human lung has a high ventilation-perfusion ratio (see Figures 5-8, 5-9 and 5-10). Therefore, the apex has a higher alveolar P_{O_2} than the base. The other choices are incorrect because the ventilation of the apex is lower than that of the base, the pH in end-capillary blood is higher because of the reduced P_{CO_2} at the apex, the blood flow is lower as already stated, and the alveoli are larger because of the regional differences of intrapleural pressure (Figure 7-8).

8. E is correct. A decreased ventilation-perfusion ratio reduces the alveolar P_{O_2} and therefore the oxygen uptake by the lung unit. The other choices are incorrect because the unit will show a decreased alveolar P_{O_2} as already stated, an increased alveolar P_{CO_2}, a change in alveolar P_{N_2} (in fact a small rise), and a reduction in the pH of end-capillary blood because of the increased P_{CO_2}.

9. D is correct. First, we calculate the ideal alveolar P_{O_2} using the alveolar gas equation. This is $P_{A_{O_2}} = P_{I_{O_2}} - P_{A_{CO_2}}/R + F$, and we ignore the small factor F. Therefore, the ideal alveolar $P_{O_2} = 149 - 48/0.8$, that is, 89 mm Hg. However, the arterial P_{O_2} is given as 49 so that the alveolar-arterial difference for P_{O_2} is 40 mm Hg.

Chapter 6

1. D is correct. Normal arterial blood has a P_{O_2} of about 100 mm Hg. The concentration of oxygen in the absence of hemoglobin is the dissolved oxygen, which is 100×0.003, or 0.3 ml $O_2 \cdot 100$ ml^{-1} blood. However, normal arterial blood contains about 15 g$\cdot$100 ml^{-1} of hemoglobin, and each gram can combine with 1.39 ml O_2. Since the oxygen saturation of normal arterial blood is about 97%, the total oxygen concentration is given by $(1.39 \times 15 \times 97/100) + 0.3$ ml $O_2 \cdot 100$ ml^{-1} blood. This is about 20.5 as opposed to the dissolved oxygen concentration of 0.3 ml $O_2 \cdot 100$ ml^{-1} blood. Therefore, the presence of hemoglobin increases the oxygen concentration about 70 times.

2. E is correct. A small amount of carbon monoxide added to blood increases its oxygen affinity, that is, it causes a leftward shift of the O_2 dissociation curve (see Figure 6-2). All the other choices reduce the oxygen affinity of hemoglobin, that is, they shift the dissociation curve to the right (see Figure 6-3).

3. E is correct. Since the solubility of oxygen is 0.003 ml $O_2 \cdot 100$ ml^{-1} blood, an arterial P_{O_2} of 2000 mm Hg will increase the concentration of the dissolved oxygen to 6 ml $O_2 \cdot 100$ ml^{-1} blood. Note that this actually exceeds the normal arterial-venous difference for the oxygen concentration.

4. D is correct. In a patient with severe anemia but normal lungs, the oxygen concentration of arterial blood will be reduced, and therefore, if the cardiac output and oxygen uptake are normal, the oxygen concentration of mixed venous blood will also be reduced. The other choices are incorrect because the arterial P_{O_2} and O_2 saturation will be normal if the patient has normal lungs, but of course the arterial oxygen concentration will be reduced, and the tissue P_{O_2} will therefore be abnormally low. Note that a patient with severe anemia usually has some increase in cardiac output, but nevertheless, the oxygen concentration of mixed venous blood will be low. As in all these questions, the one best answer is being sought, and this is clearly D. See Table 6-1 for a summary of these changes.

5. C is correct. Because the oxygen concentration of arterial blood is reduced, this must also be true of mixed venous blood, other things being equal. The other choices are incorrect. If the patient has normal lungs, the arterial P_{O_2} will be normal, but of course the oxygen concentration of arterial blood will be reduced. Carbon monoxide shifts the O_2 dissociation curve to the left, that is, it increases the oxygen affinity of the hemoglobin. Carbon monoxide has no odor, which is one reason why it is so dangerous. See Table 6-1 for the changes.

6. E is correct. Since the patient is breathing air, the inspired P_{O_2} is about 149 mm Hg. Using the alveolar gas equation, the alveolar P_{O_2} will be

about 149 – 110, that is, 39 mm Hg for an R value of 1, and even less for an R value of less than 1. This is below the stated arterial P_{O_2}, which cannot be correct. In addition, the other four choices are clearly wrong. The patient does not have a normal P_{O_2} or P_{CO_2}, and there is an acidosis rather than an alkalosis.

7. B is correct. As the first column of Figure 6-4 shows, about 90% of the CO_2 transported in the arterial blood is in the form of bicarbonate. About 5% is dissolved and another 5% is transported as carbamino compounds. The most important of these is carbaminohemoglobin.

8. C is correct. The abnormally high P_{CO_2} of 60 mm Hg and the reduced pH of 7.35 are consistent with a partially compensated respiratory acidosis. Figure 6-8A shows that if the P_{CO_2} rises to 60 mm Hg and there is no renal compensation, the pH is less than 7.3. Therefore, the patient shows some compensation. The fact that the pH has not fully returned to the normal value of 7.4 means that the respiratory acidosis is only partially compensated. The other choices are incorrect because clearly the gas exchange with the high P_{CO_2} is not normal, there is an acidosis rather than an alkalosis because the pH is reduced, and this is not a metabolic acidosis because the P_{CO} is elevated.

9. A is correct. As described in the section titled "Blood-Tissue Gas Exchange," the P_{O_2} inside skeletal muscle cells is about 3 mm Hg. The blood in the peripheral capillaries has much higher P_{O_2} values in order to enable the diffusion of oxygen to the mitochondria.

10. A is correct. There is a respiratory acidosis because the P_{CO_2} is increased to 50 mm Hg and the pH is reduced to 7.20. However, there must be a metabolic component to the acidosis because as Figure 6-8A shows, a P_{CO_2} of 50 will reduce the pH to only about 7.3 if the point moves along the normal blood buffer line. Therefore, there must be a metabolic component to reduce the pH even further. The other choices are incorrect because, as indicated above, an uncompensated respiratory acidosis would give a pH of above 7.3 for this P_{CO_2}. Clearly, the patient does not have a fully compensated respiratory acidosis because then the pH would be 7.4. There is not an uncompensated metabolic acidosis because the P_{CO_2} is increased, indicating a respiratory component. Finally, there is not a fully compensated metabolic acidosis because this would give a pH of 7.4.

11. E is correct. A is incorrect because there is no metabolic compensation. In fact, the bicarbonate concentration is abnormally high. B is incorrect because the P_{CO_2} is low, which is incompatible with a respiratory acidosis. C is incorrect because a metabolic acidosis requires an abnormally low bicarbonate concentration, which this patient does not have. D is incorrect because the patient has an acidosis, not an alkalosis. Therefore, the correct answer can be found by eliminating the other four. However, in addition, Figure 6-8A shows that there is no way that the three

given values can coexist on the diagram. Therefore, there must be a laboratory error.

12. E is correct. The reduction in the pH to 7.30 with a small reduction in the P_{CO_2} from 40 to 32 is consistent with a partially compensated metabolic acidosis. Compensation is only partial because if it was complete, the pH would be 7.4. The other choices are incorrect. This is not a respiratory alkalosis because the pH is abnormally low. When the alveolar-arterial P_{O_2} difference is calculated using the alveolar gas equation, the alveolar P_{O_2} is about 149 – 32/0.8, that is, 109 mm Hg giving a difference of 109 – 90, or 19 mm Hg. This is abnormally high. The arterial oxygen saturation will be greater than 70% because with a P_{O_2} of 90 mm Hg, the saturation will be above 90% as shown in Figure 6-1. It is true that the reduced P_{CO_2} will shift the curve slightly to the left and the increased hydrogen ion concentration will shift it slightly to the right, but the P_{O_2} is so high that the saturation must be more than 70%. Recall that with a normal oxygen dissociation curve, an arterial P_{O_2} of 40 gives an oxygen saturation of about 75%, so a P_{O_2} of 90 will certainly result in a saturation of over 70%. The sample was not mistakenly taken from a vein because then the P_{O_2} would be very much lower.

Chapter 7

1. B is correct. When the diaphragm contracts, it becomes flatter as shown in Figure 7-1. The other choices are incorrect. The phrenic nerves that innervate the diaphragm come from high in the neck, that is, cervical segments 3, 4, and 5. Contraction of the diaphragm causes the lateral distance between the lower rib margins to increase and anterior abdominal wall to move out as also shown in Figure 7-1. The intrapleural pressure is reduced because the larger volume of the chest cage increases the recoil pressure of the lung.

2. C is correct. If there is less lung, the total change in volume per unit change in pressure will be reduced. The other choices are incorrect. Compliance increases with age, filling a lung with saline increases compliance (Figure 7-5), absence of surfactant decreases compliance, and in the upright lung at FRC, inspiration causes a larger increase in volume of the alveolar at the base of the lung compared with those near the apex (Figure 7-8).

3. A is correct. The Laplace relationship shown in Figure 7-4C states that the pressure is inversely proportional to the radius for the same surface tension. Since bubble X has three times the radius of bubble Y, the ratio of pressures will be approximately 0.3:1.

4. E is correct. Surfactant is produced by type II alveolar epithelial cells as discussed in relation to Figure 7-6.

bicarbonate concentration of the CSF can affect the output of the central chemoreceptors by buffering the changes in pH.

3. B is correct. The peripheral chemoreceptors are responsive to the arterial P_{O_2}, but during normoxia, the response is small (see Figure 8-3B). The other choices are incorrect. Peripheral chemoreceptors do respond to changes in blood pH, the response to changes in P_{CO_2} is faster than is the case for central chemoreceptors, the central chemoreceptors are more important than the peripheral chemoreceptors in the ventilatory response to increased CO_2, and peripheral chemoreceptors have a very high blood flow in relation to their mass.

4. E is correct. The normal level of ventilation is controlled by the ventilatory response to CO_2. The other choices are incorrect. The ventilatory response to CO_2 is increased if the alveolar P_{O_2} is reduced, the ventilatory response depends on the peripheral chemoreceptors in addition to the central chemoreceptors, and the ventilatory response is reduced during sleep and if the work of breathing is increased.

5. A is correct. Ventilation increases greatly at high altitude in response to hypoxic stimulation of chemoreceptors. The other choices are incorrect. It is the peripheral chemoreceptors, not the central chemoreceptors that are responsible for the response. The response is increased if the P_{CO_2} is also raised. Hypoxic stimulation is often important in patients with long-standing severe lung disease who have nearly normal values for the pH of the CSF and blood. Mild carbon monoxide poisoning is associated with a normal arterial P_{O_2}, and therefore, there is no stimulation of the peripheral chemoreceptors.

6. D is correct. As Figure 8-2 shows, the most important stimulus comes from the pH of the CSF on the central chemoreceptors. The other choices are incorrect. The effect of P_{O_2} on the peripheral chemoreceptors under normoxic conditions is very small. Changes in P_{CO_2} do affect the peripheral chemoreceptors, but the magnitude is less than that for the central chemoreceptors. The effect of changes in pH on peripheral chemoreceptors under normal conditions is small, and changes in P_{O_2} do not affect the central chemoreceptors.

7. E is correct. Moderate exercise does not reduce the arterial P_{O_2}, increase the arterial P_{CO_2}, or reduce the arterial pH. The P_{O_2} of mixed venous blood does fall, but there are no known chemoreceptors that are stimulated as a result.

8. D is correct. The other choices are incorrect. The impulses travel to the brain via the vagus nerve, the reflex inhibits further inspiratory efforts if the lung is maintained inflated, the reflex is not seen in adults at small tidal volumes, and abolishing the reflex by cutting the vagal nerves in experimental animals causes slow deep breathing.

Chapter 9

1. A is correct. In some elite athletes, oxygen consumption can increase 15-fold or even 20-fold. The other choices are incorrect. The measured R value can exceed 1 at high levels of exercise because lactic acid is produced and there are very high levels of ventilation. Ventilation increases much more than cardiac output (Figure 9-13), and at low levels of exercise, little or no lactate is normally produced. During moderate levels of exercise, there is essentially no change in pH.

2. E is correct. There is a rise in oxidative enzymes in muscle cells that assists acclimatization. The other choices are incorrect. Hyperventilation is the most important feature of acclimatization, polycythemia occurs slowly, there is a leftward shift of the O_2 dissociation curve at extreme altitude because of the respiratory alkalosis, and the number of capillaries per unit volume of skeletal muscle increases with acclimatization.

3. B is correct (see Figure 9-4 for a full explanation). The other choices are incorrect. Atelectasis occurs faster during oxygen breathing than air breathing, blood flow to an atelectatic lung is reduced because of the low lung volume and perhaps hypoxic pulmonary vasoconstriction, the absorption of a spontaneous pneumothorax can be explained by the same mechanism, and the elastic properties of the lung have little effect in resisting atelectasis caused by gas absorption.

4. A is correct because decompression sickness is caused by bubbles of gas, and helium is less soluble than nitrogen. The other choices are incorrect. The work of breathing and the airway resistance are both decreased. The risk of O_2 toxicity is unchanged, but the risk of inert gas narcosis is decreased.

5. C is correct. In zero G, the deposition of inhaled particles by sedimentation is abolished. The other choices are incorrect. Both blood flow and ventilation to the apex of the lung are increased because the normal effects of gravity are abolished (see Figures. 2-7, 4-7, and 5-8). Thoracic blood volume increases because blood no longer pools in dependent regions of the body as a result of gravity. The P_{CO_2} at the apex of the lung increases because the abolition of gravity results in a reduction of the VA/Q at the apex (see Figure 5-10).

6. B is correct. Alveolar ventilation like total ventilation can increase by a factor of 10 or more. The other choices are incorrect. Heart rate, cardiac output, and the P_{CO_2} of mixed venous blood increase much less. Also, tidal volume increases much less because part of the increase in alveolar ventilation is caused by the increase in respiratory frequency.

7. C is correct. The ductus arteriosus closes (see the discussion of Figure 9-5). There is a big increase in arterial P_{O_2}, a large fall in pulmonary vascular resistance, a decreased blood flow through the foramen ovale, and very large inspiratory efforts.

Chapter 10

1. A is correct. Bronchodilators reduce airway resistance, and their efficacy can therefore be assessed by this test. The other choices are incorrect. Dynamic compression of the airways is the main factor limiting maximal expiratory flow, the flow is greatly reduced in chronic obstructive pulmonary disease but may be normal or even increased in pulmonary fibrosis, it is reduced in patients with asthma, and it is easy to perform.

2. D is correct. Loss of radial traction is one of the factors contributing to dynamic compression of the airways in COPD. The other choices are incorrect. The action of the diaphragm does not affect dynamic compression; if a bronchodilator drug is effective, it may increase the FEV; the flow is independent of expiratory effort; and increased elastic recoil does not occur in COPD although if it did, this could increase the FEV.

3. D is correct (see discussion of Figure 2-6). The other choices are incorrect. The slope of the alveolar plateau is increased in chronic bronchitis because poorly ventilated units empty later in expiration than well-ventilated units. The last exhaled gas comes from apex of the lung because of airway closure at the base, and the test is not very time consuming.

4. B is correct (see the Discussion under "Measurement of Ventilation-Perfusion Inequality" in Chapter 5). The other choices are incorrect. The ideal alveolar P_{O_2} is calculated using the arterial P_{CO_2}, and VA/Q inequality increases the alveolar-arterial P_{O_2} difference, the physiologic shunt, and the physiologic dead space.

5. B is correct. Near the end of the expiration, the expired gas comes preferentially from the apex of the lung because of airway closure at the base (see Figure 7-9). The apex of the lung has a relatively low P_{CO_2} (see Figure 5-10). The other choices are incorrect. The residual volume is much less than half of the vital capacity; if the airway is obstructed at RV and the subject relaxes, the pressure in the airways is less than atmospheric pressure (see Figure 7-11); intrapleural pressure is always less than alveolar pressure; and only the airways near the base of the lung are closed at residual volume (see Figure 7-9).

Figure Credits

Figure 1-1	From Weibel ER: *Respir Physiol* 11:54, 1970.
Figure 1-2	Scanning electron micrograph by Nowell JA, Tyler WS.
Figure 1-4	Modified from Weibel ER: *The Pathway for Oxygen.* Cambridge: Harvard University Press, 1984, p. 275.
Figure 1-6	From Maloney JE, Castle BL: *Respir Physiol* 7:150, 1969.
Figure 1-7	From Glazier JB, et al: *J Appl Physiol* 26:65, 1969.
Figure 2-1	Modified from West JB: *Ventilation/Blood Flow and Gas Exchange*, ed. 5. Oxford: Blackwell, 1990, p. 3.
Figure 4-2	From Hughes JMB, et al: *Respir Physiol* 4:58, 1968.
Figure 4-7	Redrawn from Hughes JMB, et al: *Respir Physiol* 4:58, 1968.
Figure 4-8	From West JB, et al: *J Appl Physiol* 19:713, 1964.
Figure 4-10	From Barer GR, et al: *J Physiol* 211:139, 1970.
Figure 5-2	Modified from West JB: *Ventilation/Blood Flow and Gas Exchange*, ed. 5. Oxford: Blackwell, 1990, p. 3.
Figure 5-5	From West JB: *Ventilation/Blood Flow and Gas Exchange*, ed. 5. Oxford: Blackwell, 1990.
Figure 5-6	From West JB: *Ventilation/Blood Flow and Gas Exchange*, ed. 5. Oxford: Blackwell, 1990.
Figure 5-7	From West JB: *Ventilation/Blood Flow and Gas Exchange*, ed. 5. Oxford: Blackwell, 1990.
Figure 5-8	From West JB: *Ventilation/Blood Flow and Gas Exchange*, ed. 5. Oxford: Blackwell, 1990.
Figure 5-9	From West JB: *Ventilation/Blood Flow and Gas Exchange*, ed. 5. Oxford: Blackwell, 1990.
Figure 5-11	From West JB: *Lancet* 2:1055, 1963.
Figure 5-12	Modified from West JB: *Ventilation/Blood Flow and Gas Exchange*, ed. 5. Oxford: Blackwell, 1990.
Figure 5-13	Redrawn from Wagner et al: *J Clin Invest* 54:54, 1974.
Figure 5-14	Redrawn from Wagner et al: *J Clin Invest* 54:54, 1974.
Figure 7-5	From Radford EP: *Tissue Elasticity.* Washington, DC: American Physiological Society, 1957.
Figure 7-6	From Weibel ER, Gil J. In West JB: *Bioengineering Aspects of the Lung.* New York: Marcel Dekker, 1977.
Figure 7-8	From West JB: *Ventilation/Blood Flow and Gas Exchange*, ed. 5. Oxford: Blackwell, 1990.

Figure 7-9	From West JB: *Ventilation/Blood Flow and Gas Exchange*, ed. 5. Oxford: Blackwell, 1990.
Figure 7-14	Redrawn from Pedley TJ, et al: *Respir Physiol* 9:387, 1970.
Figure 7-15	Redrawn from Briscoe WA, Dubois AB: *J Clin Invest* 37:1279, 1958.
Figure 7-17	Redrawn from Fry DL, Hyatt RE: *Am J Med* 29:672, 1960.
Figure 7-20	Modified from West JB: *Ventilation/Blood Flow and Gas Exchange*, ed. 5. Oxford: Blackwell, 1990.
Figure 8-4	From Nielsen M, Smith H: *Acta Physiol Scand* 24:293, 1951.
Figure 8-5	Modified from Loeschke HH, Gertz KH: *Arch Ges Physiol* 267:460, 1958.
Figure 9-3	From Hurtado A. In Dill DB: *Handbook of Physiology, Adaptation to the Environment*. Washington, DC: American Physiological Society, 1964.
Figure 10-5	Modified from Comroe JH: *The Lung: Clinical Physiology and Pulmonary Function Tests*, ed. 2. Chicago: Year Book, 1965.

Index

Note: Pages that followed by *f* represents figure and that followed by *t* represents table.